KEEPER OF THE WOODS

KEEPER OF THE WOODS

BY

CHESTER A. "CHET" BALLARD

ISBN: 1-58500-981-4

Library of Congress Copyright applied for.
ISBN number 0-9646070-2-6

1stbooks – rev. 2/12/00

About the Book

A Horror/thriller with a Love story, as well as lust. It is also a study of the relationship between three fathers and their sons as they face death. A real tearjerker at times.

An abandoned military base is opened to the public for hunting and motorcycle riding.

One Father takes his two sons for a last hunting trip together.

Another Father goes motorcycle riding with his son and nine friends.

What starts out as a fun weekend ends up in death and despair. They are not alone in the woods. These people are hunted down and killed by a hermit that feels that they are trespassers on his land. He knows of only one way to deal with trespassers. They must die.

**FUTURE NOVELS TO BE RELEASED BY
CHESTER A. "CHET" BALLARD**

**STALKER
DARK VISIONS
SYSTEM SHOCK
CITY OF DREAMS
LAST CHANCE
BRENNAN'S HOPE
MANIFESTATION
ALASKAN TERROR
PRESENCE OF EVIL
TASTE OF REVENGE
TALES OF VENGEANCE
SONGS OF THE NIGHT
RING OF TERROR
PRICE OF VENGEANCE
CITY UNDER SIEGE
SHATTERED GLASS**

This book is dedicated
to my son,

Sean E. Ballard,

for all the happiness
he has brought into my
life.

And to my Grandchildren

Chance Arthur Ballard
Brennan Michael Ballard
Lacy Nicole Ballard
Ashton Nicole Ballard
Makenna Elise Freeman

SPECIAL RECOGNITION
TO

J.P. Klenke, Mark and Tiffanie Morris, Joan Camp, Farah Azarnia, Farough Tolle, Phillip Lillard, Chris Ballard, April Schell, Jim Schell, Chad Ballard, Allison Lomax, Elton Ballard, Emma Ballard, Kelly Gerald, Dennis Schell, Judy Schell, Larry Daniel, Mary Daniel, John Camp, Verna Coppinger, Coreta, Ray, and Roberta Thibodeaux.

SPECIAL APPRECIATION
TO

MY LOVING WIFE

Sharon Elizabeth Ballard

She makes every day worth living.

CHAPTER 1

The headlights of the Ford pickup truck shining on the trees and the bushes that surrounded the narrow dirt road cast eerie shadows in front of the couple as they drove the winding road that led deep into the forest. The girl was sitting so close to the driver in the front seat of the truck that with each bump the truck tires hit she had to hold onto the dashboard or she would have bounced on top of him. The sound of her giggles was the only noise that pierced the silence of the moonless night.

After driving two miles down the road, the driver stopped the truck and turned off the engine and the headlights. The couple sat in the darkness for a full minute before she finally spoke.

"Well. What do we do now, Greg?" she asked him. She could barely make out his outline in the darkness.

"Give me a drink, and then we'll see," he answered as he turned the knob on the dashboard and the overhead light came on.

Darlene opened the ice chest on the floorboard beside her and took out a quart beer bottle. She took a drink from it and handed it to him. He took a long drink from the bottle and emptied it.

"You had better take it easy," she said. "That's the third bottle we've had tonight, and you drank most of them. I can't drive a stick shift, and I sure don't want you passing out on me because I'll be damned if I want to spend the night out here in these spooky woods."

"Don't worry about me. I can handle it."

"What else can you handle?" she asked him teasingly as she pulled off her shirt and threw it on the floor of the truck.

Greg's eyes almost popped from their sockets as he stared at her large breasts. He knew they were big, but he had no idea they were that big. Her nipples were standing straight out and the brown area surrounding them made them look like huge fried eggs. He grabbed one in each hand and began to rub them roughly.

1

"Hold on a minute," the girl said as she pushed his hands away. "They are not cantaloupes you are feeling to see if they are ripe. You are supposed to rub them gently. You act like these are the first breasts you have ever touched, or even seen."

Greg was glad that the light in the interior of the truck was dim. He knew his face had to be as red as a beet from blushing. He was glad because he didn't want her to know that they were the first breasts he had ever seen, except for the ones in magazines or in the porno videos he had found in his parents' bedroom.

"They aren't the only ones I've seen," he lied. "But I have to say they are the biggest. I guess the beer made me forget to be gentle."

"Greg, don't worry about it," Darlene said as she returned his hands to her breasts.

Greg did his best to muster all the self control he could summon from within him to rub her slowly and gently. He sensed that he was not doing it correctly when she began to fidget nervously.

"Let me show you," Darlene said as she put her hands on top of his and began to move his hands in a wide circle around each breast. With each movement she would shorten the circle until his hands were making small circles around her nipples. Then she took his fingers and made him pinch the tips of them lightly.

Greg let his hands go limp and let her control them totally. He watched as she began to fidget in the seat again. This time it was plain for him to see that she was enjoying it. He watched her face as she closed her eyes. Low moaning sounds emitted from her throat that grew louder as he stroked her. After a few minutes, she stopped moving his hands and pushed them away again. She scooted across the seat and leaned back on the passenger door.

"Let's get on with this," Darlene ordered as she arched her back and slid off her shorts.

Greg had to swallow a huge lump that suddenly appeared in his throat as he looked between her legs at her femininity.

2

"Well, are you just going to stare at it?" Darlene asked. "Or are you going to do something with it?"

Greg forced himself to go slow as he put his hands between her legs and began stroking.

"I can do that myself anytime," she said angrily as she grabbed him around the neck and pulled his head between her legs. "Lick it! Lick it hard!" she demanded.

Greg was getting more confused with each passing moment. He was also trying to remember everything so he would not be so inexperienced the next time. The beer began to take effect and made him dizzy . It also made it hard for him to think clearly. He tried to store everything that was happening in his mind. Rub breasts gently. Be rough other places. He tried to remember the porno films he had seen. The people in them always seemed to be rough with each other. He realized through the fog in his brain that the movies were not always like real life.

He lifted his head to take a breath and looked up at Darlene. She was rubbing both her breasts at the same time. She was apparently enjoying herself. Her eyes were rolled back in her head and she was moaning even louder now. She pushed his head back between her legs and wrapped them around his broad shoulders. Each time his tongue would touch her, she would raise off the seat and force herself even closer to his face.

Greg lost all track of time as he continued doing what she told him to do. A sound that resembled more of a scream than a moan filled the interior of the truck. Greg raised up quickly.

"Don't stop now, you bastard!" Darlene screamed at him as she pushed his head back down.

Greg continued as he had before and listened as her moans grew louder. He was glad that he had brought her out to the middle of the woods. If they had stopped near the main road, the people in the passing cars would surely have heard her.

He felt her legs tighten around him as she shuddered violently and let out a low whimper instead of a scream this time. He had read enough books to know that she had reached her climax. She pushed his head away from her and he began kissing the inside of her legs gently. She didn't have to tell him to do this. He remembered reading or seeing it somewhere. He

3

knew she liked it because she began to let loud sighs escape from her.

"What was that?" Darlene yelled as she pushed him away again and sat upright in the seat.

"What was **what**?"

"I think someone just walked past the truck," Darlene answered.

"I think you're imagining things. Who would be way out here in the middle of the night?"

"We're out here!" Darlene answered.

"Yes. But we are in a truck. Look out there. It is totally black. No one could be walking here without a flashlight. Did you see a flashlight?" Greg asked.

"No. I just saw something pass by the truck," Darlene said slowly.

"I think you had too much to drink," Greg said as he began to lower his head between her legs.

"Maybe you're right. Come up here," Darlene said as she grabbed him by his arms and pulled him on top of her.

She pressed her lips to his and slipped her tongue into his mouth. She helped him unbuckle his belt and used her feet to slide his pants down around his knees. She was going to do the same with his underwear, but he had already pulled them down and was fumbling to get inside of her. He was trying so hard that he kept missing his target.

"Wait a minute," Darlene demanded as she reached between his legs and guided him into her.

She hit her foot on the steering wheel but did not feel the pain as she wrapped her legs around his waist and forced him deep inside of her. He began to pump wildly and quickly as she rose from the seat and matched his movements. She was about to tell him to slow down when he groaned and stopped.

"Don't stop now!" she yelled.

Greg continued pumping her as quickly as he had before. He tried to shut out all the visions of her breasts and the pictures of naked women he had seen in magazines and movies that seemed to fill his memory. He couldn't do it. It took only a few more thrusts before he felt as if his brain, as well as his member

4

were both exploding. He collapsed in exhaustion on top of her and lay still.

"Don't tell me you're through!" Darlene said angrily.

"It must have been all the beer," Greg answered.

"Bullshit! It was because you are selfish," Darlene said with contempt.

"What are you complaining about? You got yours," Greg said in a loud voice. His embarrassment was beginning to turn to anger.

"You really don't know a damn thing about women, do you?" she accused.

"What are you talking about?" he asked in frustration.

Darlene pushed him off of her and sat upright in the seat. She lit a cigarette and inhaled deeply and blew it toward his face as she stared at him.

"A woman can have multiple orgasms while men usually stop after one. That's why it is important for men to hold back."

"I know that," Greg said. He had read that somewhere, too. "Just give me a few minutes, and we'll do it again."

"Do what again? You mean I can have ten more seconds of pleasure if I wait an hour or so for you to be able to get it up again? No, thank you. I think you can just take me home. I'll have to put off the second pleasure trip until another time. That is, if there is another time."

"Whatever you say," Greg said as he started the engine.

He almost screamed as he pulled the switch and the headlights illuminated the road in front of him. He could have sworn that he saw a figure of a man run across the road and disappear into the trees.

"What's the matter now?" Darlene asked as she saw the expression on his face change.

"I thought I saw someone out there," he replied.

"You are just like all men. When a woman thinks she saw something, as I did a while ago, it's our imagination. But when a man sees something, it's a real thing."

"I guess you are right," Greg agreed. "It was probably a deer or something like that."

"Maybe it was a man that saw you screwing me and got so

ashamed for you that he ran away into the woods." She felt nothing but contempt for Greg at that moment.

"There's no need for you to talk like that to me," Greg said. He was becoming angrier with each word she said.

"Here. Have another drink," she ordered. "It may help to clear your head after all the exertion you put out on that ten second sex marathon."

Greg grabbed the bottle from her hand and drank over half of it before he handed it back to her. The alcohol must have gone straight to his brain, or it was the most beer his body could stand for one night. He immediately felt dizzy and his vision blurred. He felt his stomach churning.

"**Get me the hell out of here!**" Darlene said angrily.

Greg put the truck in gear and tried to turn around. The road was too narrow so he had to back up. In his haste, or because of the effects of the beer, he misjudged the distance and backed off the road and the rear tires of the truck went into the muddy ditch. He pressed down on the accelerator, but the tires spun rapidly in the mud.

"I think we're stuck," he said as he eased his foot off the accelerator.

"We had better not be! If I'm late my father will kill me," she answered.

"*What do you propose I do*? Do you see a telephone in this truck? If you do, then you have my permission to call for a tow truck."

"Brad had one in his car," she whined.

Greg knew who she was talking about. He was the guy she had dated for two years. Brad was also the richest kid in school.

"Yes, I know. Brad had a lot of things. He had money and a fancy car with a telephone."

"That's not all he had that you don't. He had stamina. He lasted a lot longer than you did when we were having sex," Darlene snarled.

"Then why didn't you keep dating Brad? Never mind, I remember. Didn't he start dating that new girl in school? The tall blonde with the legs that seemed to go on forever?"

"Brad loves me. He just was infatuated with her. Once he

gets what he wants from her and realizes what he gave up, he'll come back to me," Darlene informed him.

"Is that why you went out with me? To make him jealous and make him face that reality sooner?" Greg asked.

"That's part of it," she admitted. "The other reason is because I have never screwed a big football star like you. I always heard that a football star is supposed to be a big stud. I guess I heard wrong on that one."

"Let's just forget it. I'll see if I can get us out of here and we'll forget this whole night ever took place," Greg said in frustration.

"I only wish I could," Darlene mumbled.

Greg got out of the truck and went to the rear. He cursed as he tripped and fell into the mud. He could hardly see in the darkness. The light from inside the cab of the truck did not cast any light behind it. He walked across the road and stood with his back to the glare of the headlights. He saw the logs lying at the edge of the woods and pulled two of them back to the rear of the truck. He shoved one of them behind the tire and the other one in front of it. He was so engrossed in his work that he did not hear the footsteps of the shadowy figure that walked slowly toward the truck.

The figure was only thirty feet away from Greg when he stepped on a fallen tree branch, and it made a loud snapping sound. Greg stopped and stared into the darkness. The figure stood perfectly still and blended in with the woods.

Greg strained his eyes and his ears. He had heard something, or had he? He couldn't be sure. He was half drunk and **all the way** angry at Darlene and himself. He was angry at Darlene for degrading him, and even angrier at himself for letting her get away with it. When he did not hear another sound for a few seconds, he returned to his work. He kicked the log hard and wedged it underneath the tire of the truck. Then he went around and got back into the truck. The figure began to move toward the truck again.

"Maybe we can get out of here now," Greg said as he slid behind the steering wheel.

"You're covered with mud," Darlene said as soon as she saw him. "And it stinks!"

"Don't worry about it. If this works, you won't have to be around me for much longer."

Greg floored the accelerator again, but the tires still spun freely. He put the truck in reverse and backed up, then shoved it in first gear again. The truck was still stuck in the mud.

****

The figure came nearer to the truck with each step he took. He was only ten feet away now and could see the couple's faces plainly. He could tell from the young man's expression that he was angry. The figure knew the reason, too. He had stood outside the truck and watched as they had performed their act of coupling. He could have gotten both of them more easily then, but he didn't. He had decided to let them have their pleasure. After all, it would be the last they ever had. He remembered the one time he had tried coupling. That was many years ago. It had not been very pleasurable to him, although it was not unpleasurable, either. The act itself was not so bad. It was the aftermath that made him swear to never do it again. The woman had accused him of getting her pregnant and had insisted that he leave his woods and get a job to take care of the baby. He could have never left his woods. The woods were his home. He had spent most of his life here in peace and harmony. The only reason he had ventured out that time was so he could experience the act of coupling. He had watched the animals do it at certain times of the year. He had sensed that his season had come, too. The mistake he had made was staying with the woman after he had coupled with her. Animals were smarter. Most of them would couple, then separate. That is what he should have done. The woman had turned bitter after they had coupled. She let him stay with her, but he had to work like a mule around that rundown farm. She demanded to know where he was every minute. She didn't want to couple anymore, either.

He moved another few steps closer to the truck. He was close enough now to hear their voices clearly.

****

"I thought you said that would work," Darlene said.

"It still might," Greg said as he continued putting the truck in reverse, then forward. The truck rocked back and forth several times.

****

The figure continued toward the truck. He carried a long, oak stick that could have served as a walking stick if it had not been six feet long and eight inches in diameter. He took a few more steps and was almost within reach of the door handle. He would pull the girl out first and throw her into the mud. If she ran away, it wouldn't matter. She could not hide from him for long... not in his woods. Then he would take care of the boy.

****

Greg continued rocking the truck back and forth. He was quickly becoming discouraged. He was almost convinced that the only thing he was accomplishing was ruining his tires and wasting his gas. He was just about to resign himself to the reality that they were going to be stranded in these woods for the rest of the night. He could not count on anyone coming to look for them when they did not arrive home on time. No one would ever think of looking for them here. He had driven fifty miles from their home to get here. Greg didn't want to take any chance of being disturbed when he made love for the first time.

****

The figure took several more steps and grabbed the door handle of the truck. The smell of the smoke from the spinning tires filled his nostrils. He lifted up on the door handle at the exact second the tires got enough traction from the logs and went speeding from the ditch.

****

It took all of Greg's strength to control the truck as the tires broke free from the mud and rolled back onto the road and headed toward the trees on the other side of the road. He turned the wheel just in time to avoid hitting a large pine tree. Greg heard Darlene scream. He grabbed her as the door on her side swung open, and she almost fell out of the truck. He guided the truck back onto the road and slowed down.

"I hope you are happy now. At least we won't have to spend the night here," he said.

"I'm not as happy as I could be," Darlene said softly.

Greg noticed the change in the tone of her voice and looked at her with a puzzled look.

"Stop the truck," she said. She **had to get her way** or else.

"What is it?" Greg asked as he slammed on the brakes.

"I want to make love again," she answered.

"**What**?"

"I want you to make love to me again," she repeated.

"I thought you said I stunk from the mud," Greg argued.

"You do. But for some strange reason it turns me on."

Greg eyed her closely. She was still naked. For an instant he was ready to crawl on top of her and take her again. For some reason the feeling faded as quickly as it had come. He saw her for what she really was. She was just like every woman he had seen in the magazines and on the videos.

"Darlene, you are a real slut."

"I know. But I don't care. I want you to screw me again," she begged.

"What would your parents say if you came home covered with mud?" Greg asked.

"I don't care what they would say."

"You said I didn't last long enough the first time," he replied.

"You really are naive, aren't you? Most men don't last very long the first time they make love. It takes practice. So, let's practice, Greg."

"I don't think so," he said slowly.

"Are you turning me down? I've never been turned down for anything in my life!"

"I know. Darlene, you are a spoiled brat. Your parents give you everything you want."

"Not everything," she argued.

"What did you want and did not receive?"

"I wanted a new car. My other one is already two years old, and they won't get me a new one," she complained.

"Poor little girl," Greg said with contempt.

"I'm not poor!" Darlene yelled. "You're poor!!"

It was like a light had been turned on in his head. Greg began to understand a lot of things now.

"You want your parents to know I screwed you, don't you? You want to make them feel ashamed because you slept with a poor boy from the wrong side of town. You didn't want to go out with me just to make Brad jealous. You also wanted to get back at your parents for not getting you a new car." Greg felt so betrayed.

"So what if those reasons are correct? What difference should it make to you? You are getting what you want. You are getting something you've never had before."

Greg stared at her in stunned silence. He could hardly believe that she was admitting it.

"Come on now, Greg. Did you really think you could hide the fact that you had never had sex before?"

"I had better get you home. We'll be late if we don't leave now."

"It's nothing to be ashamed of, Greg. That is as long as no one else knows about it."

"What do you mean by that?" he asked.

Darlene reached across the seat and turned the ignition key off.

"I mean, no one has to know that you were a virgin as long as I get what I want," Darlene offered.

"Let's get this straight, Darlene. You want me to screw you again and get mud all over you?"

"I think you are beginning to understand," Darlene said as she put her hands between his legs and squeezed him

.

****

The figure stood in the middle of the road and shook his fist at the truck as it went down the road. Two more seconds and he would have at least had the girl out of the truck.

He stopped shaking his fist and smiled with a face that was wrinkled and as tough as leather from being constantly exposed to the elements.

The night wind contained a blustery chill that would have made any normal man shiver, but it had no effect on him. The torn ragged coat and frayed hat he wore offered very little protection, yet he felt no discomfort. The years he had spent in these woods had made him almost immune to everything except the harshest weather.

He looked down the road and could barely see the bright glow of the truck's taillights. They were stopping again. Maybe he would have enough time to reach them before they left this time.

****

Greg pulled her hand from between his legs and pushed it away.

"I said **no**!" Greg yelled.

"If you don't do it again, you will be sorry," Darlene told him.

"What is that supposed to mean?" Greg asked.

"I'll tell everyone that you couldn't even get it up."

"You wouldn't dare!" Greg replied in horror.

"Why don't you try me and see?"

Greg looked deeply into her eyes. He could tell from her expression that she was not bluffing. He wondered how he could ever show his face at school again if she did tell everyone her lies. He would have to change schools. That would cause him to lose his scholarship, and there was no way he could pay for college. He looked at her body again. It held no excitement for him at all now.

"All right," he said slowly. "But let's make it quick."

"We already did it that way. I want it to last this time."

"Whatever," Greg answered as he unzipped his pants and pulled them down around his knees. He did it more slowly than he had the first time, when his whole body was consumed with passion.

Darlene grabbed him again. He was surprised when his member did not get an erection. He thought about how things could change so quickly. An hour ago he would have done anything to get her to touch him. Now he was not even aroused when she did it.

"Don't worry. I can get it up," Darlene said as she put her head in his lap.

It took only a few seconds for her actions to take their effect on Greg's body. He felt his passion and desire to have sex with her returning.

Darlene pulled him to the other side of the truck and straddled him. She moved back and forth on him as he met each of her thrusts with the same willingness. He felt her begin to shudder as she had before and make the same loud moaning sounds. She stopped and lay her head on his chest and closed her eyes.

"That wasn't so bad, was it?" she asked.

"I guess not."

"Good. Now let's get out of here," Darlene ordered.

"No way," Greg said as he pushed her back down on the seat. "I'm not finished yet."

"I'm ready to go now," Darlene demanded.

"I'm not," Greg said as he spread her legs and shoved himself into her again.

He pumped her hard and fast with a vengeance that could only be satisfied by making her squirm and suffer for all the humiliating things she had said to him. He would pull himself almost all the way out of her, then slam forward again and again. Before long she was almost screaming from the pleasure that racked her body.

After a while, he could tell that her cries of pleasure were changing to cries of pain. This did not stop him. He continued pounding himself into her relentlessly. He was going to make sure that she could not truthfully tell anyone that he did not last long enough for her. She would be so sore and walk so oddly that she would have a hard time convincing anyone.

****

The figure could see the young man through the back window of the truck. He knew where the girl was, and he knew that they were coupling again. He wished that he could warn this young man of the dangers he faced if he did not couple and run away. That danger was much worse than the danger Greg would face if they coupled long enough for him to reach the truck. He forced his legs to hurry and carry his six-foot, lanky frame to the truck.

****

Greg continued his pounding as he looked down at Darlene. Her eyes were closed. There was no reaction from her at all. She had passed out. He withdrew from her without satisfying himself and shook her gently. She still showed no sign of movement. He pulled his pants up, grabbed the beer bottle and took a short drink from it. He poured the rest in Darlene's face. If she wanted her parents to suffer for her slumming, she would be happy when she went home reeking of stale beer.

Darlene coughed as she regained consciousness and sat up in the seat.

"**Damn you!**" she screamed at him. Darlene wondered how he could be so stupid.

"What's the matter now? I gave you what you wanted."

"I'm going to be sore tomorrow," she said as she rubbed herself.

"I know."

****

The man looked ahead at the truck as he walked. They were arguing. He was right. All humans argued after they coupled. It was too late to warn the youth now. He increased his pace of approach toward the truck. It was too late to warn either of them about anything. He hoped they would argue for at least another minute or two. Then they would never argue again.

****

"You're never satisfied, are you?" Greg asked with a laugh. "First time I don't last long enough, and the second time I lasted too long."

"Let's just get out of here," Darlene said as she slid away from him and sat by the door on the passenger side.

"That's fine by me," Greg said as he started the truck, put it into first gear, and began to roll slowly forward.

****

The figure had barely reached the rear of the truck when it began to roll forward. He stopped. They would get away this time, but he would get them if they ever came back. He would be here waiting for them.

****

Greg had driven only fifty feet when Darlene started again.

"I'm still going to tell everyone you were not worth a damn," she said.

"Tell them what you want. They won't believe you!" Greg yelled.

"Some of them will believe what I say."

Greg knew she was right. He slammed on the brakes and reached across her and opened the door of the truck.

"**Get out!**" he said.

"What?" she asked suddenly.

"I said that I want you to get out. I'm sick of listening to your bitching, and I'm sick of looking at you," Greg added.

"You can't leave me out here in the middle of nowhere," Darlene said in disbelief.

"You don't think so? Just watch me," Greg said and pushed her out the door. The truck rolled forward and then stopped.

"I didn't think you had the balls to leave me out here," Darlene said as she ran to the truck and stood by the door.

"I just wanted to give you your clothes. I didn't want you to catch cold," Greg said as he threw the shirt and shorts in her face and drove quickly down the road.

The door slammed from the force of his takeoff. He looked in his rearview mirror and caught a quick glimpse of her running behind the truck. His eye also caught something else. It looked like a large shadow coming up behind her.

Greg shook that feeling from his mind. He was seeing things, just as they both had earlier. She would be safe for a few minutes. He was not going to leave her out in the woods. He would wait a few minutes and put the truck in reverse to pick her up. She would be more agreeable then. She would probably tell her lies to anyone who would listen when she got home, but he would deal with that when the time came.

****

"You bastard! I'll get you for this!" Darlene screamed as she stood in the middle of the road in total darkness.

She shivered as she stepped into her shorts and tried to pull her shirt over her head. If she had known she would be standing outside, she would have worn warmer clothes. She strained her eyes to see any sign of the truck lights . Her eyes gradually became accustomed to the night. She could see the shapes of the trees, but she did not see any lights. She did not doubt that he would return for her. She only wished it would be soon.

As she looked slowly around her, Darlene began to make out many shapes. There were many trees on each side of the road. She began to see the bushes and tall weeds that grew where the trees were sparse. An eerie feeling that she was being watched sent cold chills up and down her spine. She turned her head slowly and looked behind her. It took only a moment for her eyes to focus on the shadowy figure that stood less than ten feet away from her. It stood so perfectly still that for a fleeting instant she thought it was a tree in the middle of the road. Terror began to creep into her as she realized the shadowy figure was that of a man.

"Greg, is that you?" she asked softly as the figure took slow, deliberate steps toward her.

The shadowy figure made no sound as it drew nearer and nearer to her. The man was too tall and much too thin to be Greg.

"Who are you? What do you want?" Darlene felt so frightened.

The figure came closer.

As much as she hated to turn her back to the figure, Darlene forced herself to run down the dark road. She had taken a few steps when she felt the mud seeping into her shoes and settling between her toes. She had run off the road in the darkness and gotten into the ditch. She struggled to free herself, but the thick mud was like quicksand. As soon as she would release one foot, her other one would then be stuck. Both of her shoes came off in the thick, gooey mud. She struggled even harder as she heard the faint footsteps coming toward her. Within seconds she could hear him breathing. He was standing over her.

"Don't fight the mud, my dear," he said in an almost pleasant voice.

"What? **Who are you**?" she cried.

"That is not important. First, we have to get you out of that mud," he replied. The man's soothing voice calmed her, and she was not so afraid of him anymore.

"I can't get out. I'm stuck."

"Sure you can. Just pull one of your feet out slowly and put it near the side of the ditch. The earth is firmer there. Then pull the other one out the same way. Be sure to put most of your weight on the foot on solid ground."

Darlene did exactly as he said. She could feel the suction of the mud break loose as she pulled her foot out. Then she pulled the other one out and stepped back in the middle of the road.

"Thank you, whoever you are," she said.

"You are welcome."

"The guy I was with left me out here," Darlene announced.

"I know," he said softly.

"How do you know?"

"That is not really important, either," he answered.

"He left me out here because I wouldn't have sex with him," Darlene quickly added.

"Why do you want to lie to me?" the man demanded to know.

"I'm not lying."

"Yes, you are...I've been watching you since you came into my woods," the man explained.

Darlene felt the calmness leaving and the fear returning that she had felt when she first saw him standing on the road. She knew now that she had not imagined seeing something.

"You were standing by the truck earlier," Darlene said with fear.

"Close enough to know what was going on."

"Then you know he will be back for me," Darlene replied.

"Of course, he'll come back. Not even the cruelest animal would leave someone out here in the cold. Greg doesn't seem like an animal."

"How do you know his name?" Darlene asked.

"I know everything that goes on in my woods, Darlene."

"We didn't mean to trespass. Greg said that this property belonged to the United States Government. He said it was an abandoned military base that was once used for training and war games."

"He was only half right. The army did use it for their training exercises, but it did not belong to them. It never did. It belongs to me," the man replied.

"Well, I'm sorry. We didn't know."

"There's no harm done. You didn't hurt a single tree or flower in my woods," he agreed.

18

"I'm glad to hear that. As soon as Greg comes to his senses he'll come back and get me, and we'll leave your property."

The man answered, "I have no doubts that he will come back for you. But I'm afraid you can't leave."

"What are you saying?"

"I'm saying that you can't leave. You trespassed when you came here. Just like me, you belong to the woods now. You can never leave again."

"We'll see about that," Darlene said as she turned to run.

The man grabbed her by the hair and pulled her backwards toward him. He put his right hand over her face and the left one behind her head and held her tightly.

Darlene began to struggle but the old man's grip tightened with every move she made. She decided that it would be better not to fight him. She forced herself to become still. The old man relaxed his hold on her slightly, but she knew he still had control.

"You have offended me and the woods by wanting to leave. You have saddened even the lowliest creature in my forest," he reprimanded her.

"I change my mind. I want to stay here," Darlene said in the softest voice she could.

Darlene realized this man was crazy. Her only hope would be to bide her time until Greg returned. He was a lot stronger than this old man, and he could easily beat the hell out of him.

"I don't believe you, Darlene. I think you are lying to save yourself. I don't think you want to stay in my woods any longer than you have to."

"I swear I do!" Darlene insisted.

"If you are not lying, then you will be happy to know that you are going to stay in my woods forever. *You will stay here for eternity*."

Darlene heard the faint sound of the truck coming down the road. She listened as the sound grew louder and louder. She could barely see the backup lights when she felt the tugging on her neck.

The old man twisted her head sharply and after a loud cracking sound, Darlene's body went limp in his hands.

****

Greg slowly backed the truck down the road. He had no idea how far he had driven after pushing her from the truck. He had been so angry he had not paid attention. He was not angry anymore. He was tired and hung over. The alcohol had left his system, but its effects had lingered on. All he wanted to do now was to get home and go to bed and put this night behind him forever. He searched the driver's side of the road for Darlene. He must have driven farther than he thought he had. He was disappointed that he did not see her running down the dark road in sheer panic from the sounds of the night. He stopped the truck and listened closely. It was strangely silent. He did not even hear the sounds of an owl or a bullfrog. He had gone hunting with his father many times in the woods at night and remembered that there had always been many sounds. He backed down the road another quarter of a mile, then stopped. He knew he had not left her this far behind. He put the truck in gear and drove slowly as he watched the side of the road. He stopped again when he saw the logs sticking out of the mud in the ditch. This was where the truck had become stuck. He tried to remember about how far he had driven after he had freed the truck until he put her out.

Greg drove even more slowly as he searched the road ahead of him. His anger was returning. Darlene was probably hiding behind a tree watching him search for her. She was mean enough to let him worry even though she was scared to be alone. His anger grew until it reached the point where he was ready to play her game. He ought to leave her out here all night. That would teach her a lesson. Greg knew as soon as the thought crossed his mind that he couldn't do that to her, no matter how much he despised her at this very moment. As he scanned the road ahead of him, he tried to remember why he had been attracted to her in the first place. The answer was not long in coming. It was simple, lust. He had wanted her the first time he had seen her. He knew she was a bitch. That only made him want her more. He began to understand how powerful an emotion lust was. It had made him have sex with her the first time because he wanted to receive pleasure and give her pleasure. But the second time he had sex with her was born of a different kind of lust. That lust wanted him to make her suffer, to feel pain. He wondered what kind of a person he was because he got more pleasure from the second time he had sex with her than he did the first. He decided that when his head cleared and his stomach settled, he would give some serious thought to the entire situation.

Another thought crossed his mind as he scanned the road ahead of him and saw nothing. Maybe she had been hiding behind a tree and watched him drive past then ran to the main road. Of course, that had to be it. She was probably laughing her ass off at this very moment because he was riding around looking for her. She had plenty of time to make it back to the main road by now.

He pressed the accelerator and headed back to the main road. He slammed on his brakes and stopped when he saw the shirt lying in the middle of the road. Had it been there before? Could he have overlooked it? He was looking behind him when he passed this spot.

Greg put the truck in neutral and had barely opened the door when he heard the loud, crashing sound of breaking glass. The shock and force of the shattering windshield sent him reeling backwards against the seat, and his head slammed into the back glass and knocked him out. His head fell forward against his chest.

When he opened his eyes, Greg immediately saw the thousands of tiny fragments of glass that covered his lap. He raised his head slowly and was staring into the face of Darlene. Her mouth was wide open, and her eyes had a cold stare. He knew she was dead. He shook his head and tried to think. Did he run over her? That answer came immediately. He was stopped when the glass was broken. Someone had thrown her through the windshield. **But who**? That question was answered quickly, too.

Greg felt the tug on his arm and turned just in time to see the tall man lunge at him with a long stick. There was no room and no time for him to avoid the attack. He felt a small pain as the pointed end of the stick penetrated his chest. He felt the warm liquid as it flowed from the corners of his mouth. His eyes looked forward involuntarily and stared directly into the eyes of Darlene. He coughed once as the liquid stopped flowing and collected in his throat. Then he did not cough again, and his eyes could not see Darlene anymore, either.

CHAPTER 2

The man stood next to the fire inside his shelter and warmed his hands as he watched through the doorway as the night slowly faded away. The firelight cast a glow over him, and he was not a shadowy figure any longer.

He had disposed of the truck and taken care of the bodies of the two young people. No one would ever find the truck, and in a few days there would not be a trace left of the people. He, and the creatures of his woods, would see to that.

The man felt no remorse for his actions of the previous night. He felt no sympathy for the victims either. The world was full of victims. His father had been a victim many years ago. His father had been a victim of the Federal Government. They had taken his land away from him. The bureaucrats from Washington had told his father that it was their right to purchase any land that would suit their purpose for the safety of the United States. Sure, they had paid his father for the land, but his father was a man of principles. He didn't believe that money could buy everything. His father had grieved so much over the loss of his land that he had committed suicide. He had buried his father on his beloved land. He had placed a large wooden marker next to the grave that read simply

"Thomas M. Golden, Sr.

He died defending his woods."

That made him, Thomas M. Golden, Jr., a victim, too. He had lost his father, but not his woods. He had lived in these woods since he was fifteen. He had come back the day he buried his father, and except for the short time he had left to couple, he had lived here since that day. All those years he had avoided the soldiers as they played their silly war games. He stood by and watched as they cut down trees and built concrete bunkers to hide under as they tossed their dangerous grenades that killed the animals and trees in the woods everywhere they exploded. He watched in anger as the soldiers built a fence that surrounded the entire three thousand acres they claimed were theirs. He had been patient because he knew one day they would grow tired of the land, and they would leave. Then he could live in peace. He could find the solace in the woods that his father and he had felt so long ago. That day had come three years ago. The soldiers had left and locked the twelve foot tall gate that blocked the only road leading into his woods.

Two weeks ago two of the soldiers had returned and tore down the gate,leaving the road wide open for anyone to pass through. That had not bothered him at the time, because this area was so isolated he didn't think anyone would come in. Last night he had been proved wrong. The young couple had violated his sanctuary. Thomas Golden knew that there would be others who would come. He made up his mind to deal with them in the same way he had dealt with the couple last night. He would not do as he did with the girl. He would not give them the choice to live and stay. They were not worthy of living in his woods. They would not find life in his woods. They would know only death.

Thomas buttoned his coat and pulled his collar up around his neck as he stepped from the warmth of his shelter. The cold wind blew over him. He knew instinctively that this was going to be a particularly brutal winter. The low hanging clouds in the overcast sky told him that there would be a lot of rain this winter, too. The leaves had begun falling and the huge stately oaks that inhabited his woods were almost bare from the loss of their leaves. The ground beneath his feet and all around him was covered with millions of brown needles that had been shed from the many pine trees. The absence of the bright colors and the movement of many small and large animals in his woods did not bother him. The leaves would return in the Spring and bring new life. Beauty would surround him once again. That was the way life was in the woods.

Thomas began to walk down one of the many trails that he knew well toward the main road. He had to make his rounds to ensure that everything was as it should be in his domain.

He had not gone down the trail very far when he heard the snarling just ahead of him. The noise of the animal did not cause him to slow his stride in the least. He feared very little in his woods. A few more steps and he stood face to face with the source of the sound. He stopped. A huge, gray wolf had managed to catch a small rabbit. He could tell just by looking into the hungry gaze of the wolf that he was old. The wolf was not as fast as he once was, and he had to settle for much smaller game than he was used to.

As he took a step closer, the wolf stopped eating its quarry, and tensing his hind legs, lowered his head. The wolf never took his eyes off the man. A low growl was sent out to the man as a warning that he was not willing to share his meager breakfast with anyone.

"Don't worry. I have no intention of taking your food. You caught it, and you deserve to eat it."

The growling continued from the wolf, but it lost some of its intensity as soon as the man spoke.

"You look like you need it more than I do, anyway," Thomas said. "Look how skinny you are."

The man and the wolf stared at each other. The man noticed that the wolf only had one eye. It was probably a result of a fight with a larger wolf, or maybe even a badger. There was no way for the man to know. The forest was a dangerous place that was filled with the sounds of survival every day. It was also filled with the pain of death. Only the strong could survive in the woods. The wolf's hunger was stronger than his concern about the old man standing in front of him. He began to rip his teeth into the rabbit once again.

"I ought to take you home with me," Thomas told the wolf. "I could hunt for you, and you could enjoy what time you have left in your life in the woods. You have earned a rest."

Thomas had not expected any answer. And he did not get one as he stepped around the wolf and left him to his feeding.

He continued walking through the woods and marveled at his surroundings. The beauty of the woods never failed to amaze him. He listened intently to the sounds of the animals. He heard squirrels barking, wings fluttering, and off in the distance he could hear the sound of a fish jumping in a pond. Everything about the woods brought a smile to his face and thrilled him to his very soul.   The one thing that made him happier than anything else was that he could walk through his woods and not have to see or listen to another human being. Other people did not understand the woods, and that lack of understanding caused them to abuse the woods and all of the creatures in it.

The clanking sound of a truck pulling a large trailer distracted him from his enjoyment of the morning. He stepped behind a tree and watched as the truck turned off the main road onto the small gravel road that led into the woods and came to a stop thirty feet in front of him. Two men got out of the truck.

"Are you sure they will be all right out here in the woods, Jimmy?" one of them asked.

"They will be fine, Bill. In fact, everything will be perfect."

"Okay. As long as you're sure. We went to a lot of trouble to steal these cows. I don't want to lose them," Bill argued.

"We won't lose them. We sure can't put them in with our herd. This is the one place that the Sheriff would never dream of looking for them."

"I guess you're right. But what if they get lost in the woods?"

Bill fretted.

"They won't get lost! They will be here every morning."

"How do you know that, Jimmy?"

"Because we are going to leave some hay here today. These dumb animals will be standing at this very spot every morning waiting for us to bring them their food."

"And when the Sheriff stops looking for them, we can sell them."

"Now you're getting the idea, Bill."

Thomas watched from behind the tree as the two men removed the gate of the trailer and the cows lumbered out one at a time. He noticed that there was also a large bull among the herd. He was glad to see the cows in his forest. Some of his animals, like the old wolf he had seen on the way here, could feed on them easily. But he did not like the idea of these men coming into his woods every day. He stepped from behind the tree as the last cow was unloaded from the trailer.

"Don't ever come into my woods again!" he roared to the two men.

Jimmy and Bill looked in the direction from which the voice

had come. They saw a tall old man wearing a heavy, ragged coat and a floppy hat. The old man also carried a huge stick. The expression in the old man's eyes filled them both with a sense of dread.

"Who are you?" Jimmy asked as he pushed his fear aside.

"That doesn't matter. Get out!" Thomas ordered.

"The hell we will. If you think you are going to steal these cows from us, you're crazy!" Bill yelled.

The sound of Thomas Golden's laughter filled the woods as he ran toward the two men. As he approached them, Bill pulled a knife from the scabbard at his side and lunged toward the old man. Thomas stepped to one side, the knife barely missing his stomach.

"Both of you will die now!" Thomas screamed as he brought his stick crashing down on Bill's head. He turned and saw the one called Jimmy frozen in place. A look of fear covered his face.

"I'm going," Jimmy said. "I won't come back, either."

The old man did not say a word as he swung his stick again with all of his strength at Jimmy. The blow killed him instantly.

Thomas poked the two men to make sure their was no sign of life before he drove the truck and trailer farther down the road until he came to a large pond. As he got out of the truck, he moved the shift lever to drive and watched as the truck and trailer went down the embankment and disappeared into the murky water of a large pond.

Thomas still carried the large stick as he returned for the bodies of the two men. He was the king of these woods, and the stick would be his scepter. Anyone who trespassed in his woods would suffer the consequences.

CHAPTER 3

Arthur Billings and his wife Elizabeth stood in the living room of their two-story house, surrounded by a dozen friends and relatives. It was five o'clock Christmas Eve and Elizabeth was scurrying around making sure everyone had plenty to eat. Arthur held his two of his granddaughters and watched his wife. She was a slender woman who bore no distinguishing signs of having borne three children. She certainly did not look like a grandmother. She was slim, and her sandy blond hair was cut short in the back and long on one side. It flowed to one side of her face and covered one of her beautiful blue eyes.

As Arthur carried his granddaughters to the bedroom to check on his grandson and other granddaughter who were sleeping, he stopped in front of the full-length mirror. He didn't bear much resemblance to any other grandfather he had ever seen, either. Arthur was five-foot-six inches tall and even though he had been a computer programmer for twelve years, he still retained the stockiness and some of the muscles he had built up from his years of working construction. He carried the girls effortlessly back to the living room. He stood in front of the large picture window and looked down the street. As if she could read his thoughts, Elizabeth came over and stood beside him.

"He'll be here," she whispered.

"Who?" he asked.

"*You know who.* Sean, your son."

"And how do you know I was looking for him?"

"**Because I know you.** You want your family here on Christmas Eve."

"Am I that predictable?"

"For me you are. I have been married to you for twenty-five years, remember? Now sit down and enjoy yourself. Sean called and said he would be late."

"Sean is always late," Arthur mumbled to himself.

"I heard that," Elizabeth said as she walked away.

Arthur walked across the room and sat down on the hearth in

front of the fireplace. Someone, Arthur didn't even notice who, came and took the girls from his arms and carried them into the bedroom. They had both fallen asleep. He shut out the noise of the many conversations around him.

"Sean just called. He said to wait under the carport for him," Elizabeth shouted from the next room.

Arthur noticed the change in the festivities as the room grew silent.

"All right, what's going on?" Arthur asked.

"You'll see. Let's go outside and wait for Sean," Mark answered.

Mark Helms was a good friend of Sean's. He was tall and of medium build and had such a friendly personality that everyone liked him the moment they met him.

Arthur walked through the dining room and stepped through the door that led to the carport. Everyone in the room followed him.

"What now?" Arthur asked as he leaned against the car.

Before anyone could answer him, he heard the roar of an engine. Arthur knew immediately who was coming down the driveway. It was J.P. Keller. He was Sean's roommate and the best friend he had in the world. He drove a little sports car in which he had put an engine that was three times bigger than the original. It made an unmistakable sound as it came to a stop, and J.P. got out.

J.P. was a tall, thin man of twenty-five. He was a nice person and the oldest of Sean's friends, but Arthur had the feeling that he didn't trust anyone. Unlike Sean's other friends, J.P. never ate when he was over. He always politely refused. J.P. was the person responsible for getting Sean interested in dirt riding on motorcycles. Sean had bought himself a dirt bike, and they had been going riding for the past few weekends.

"Sean will be here in a minute," J.P. said as he walked under the carport.

"Merry Christmas, J.P.," Arthur said as he extended his hand.

"Merry Christmas, Mr. Billings."

"What is Sean up to now?" Arthur asked.

30

"He'll be here in a minute," J.P. answered.

"Why doesn't anyone want to tell me anything?" Arthur asked.

"Because it's supposed to be a surprise," Elizabeth answered.

"Do **you** know what it is?"

"Yes, but I'm not going to tell you."

"I guess I'll have to wait then," Arthur mumbled.

"You got that right!" J.P. said.

Arthur was just about to ask something else when he heard another sound coming down the driveway. This was a low whining sound. Arthur knew that it came from a motorcycle. He went to the driveway and watched as Sean pulled off the street and drove up to him. Sean was dressed in a bright red Santa Claus costume, including the beard and black boots.

"Merry Christmas, Dad," he said as he killed the engine and handed the key to Arthur.

Arthur took the key and rubbed it between his fingers. He had given up his last motorcycle twenty three years ago, the day his oldest son was born. He looked at the red Honda 125 MR dirt bike. He brushed a tear from his eye and hugged Sean around his neck tightly.

"Thanks, Sean," Arthur said with a lump in his throat.

"Thank J.P., too. He did most of the work. He practically rebuilt the motor on it."

"Thank you, too, J.P., very much," Arthur said as he reached to shake his hand.

"The hell with that," J.P. said as he brushed Arthur's hand away and hugged him. "This is Christmas. I guess I can hug you once a year."

Arthur was surprised again. J.P. had never shown any sign of affection before. Arthur had just assumed that J.P. didn't care much for him. He guessed now that he had assumed wrong. J.P. was much too complex a person to figure out that easily.

"That's not all of the surprise," Sean said.

"What more can there be?" Arthur asked.

"Next weekend, on New Year's Eve, we are all going to go riding at Camp Leder. We are going to camp out Friday night.

31

J.P.'s dad is going to let him use the Suburban. It's big enough for all three of us to sleep in. And Mark and a bunch of other people are going to meet us there the next morning. We will have a whole crowd of us riding together."

"What is Camp Leder?" Arthur inquired.

"It's an old military base that they closed down a few years ago. They just reopened it to the public for dirt bike riders. There are old abandoned bunkers all over the place."

"I don't know if I can handle that. I haven't ridden a motorcycle in over twenty years. And don't forget, I'm an old man now. I'm a grandfather," Arthur said as he pointed to the two little girls who had awakened in all the excitement and were brought outside.

"You are only forty-three. The only reason you have grandkids is because you started having your own kids early," Sean said.

"And we'll both help you get back into the habit of riding a motorcycle," J.P. said.

"Where is this place?" Arthur asked.

"About a hundred and twenty miles from here," Sean answered. "You are going to love it. It's got fifty foot hills to climb with your bike and there are hundreds of trails through the woods to ride on. It would take a month to ride on all the trails. In fact, we could spend a lifetime there."

****

The Ford Explorer left the dirt road and headed straight across the small hills, bouncing its occupants around until it stopped in the middle of a small clearing.

James Foster got out and immediately began giving orders to his two teenage sons, Jack and John.

"Unload the tent. It will be dark soon, and I want to have a fire going in an hour. I'm getting hungry."

The two boys did not need to be told twice. They opened the back door of the vehicle, and in less than thirty minutes, had the tent up and a fire going.

"Didn't I tell you boys that this would be a great way to

spend New Years?" he asked as he pointed to the woods that surrounded their camp.

"You sure did, Dad," Jack answered.

"I'll bet there are at least a hundred deer watching us right now. In fact, I think I just saw one of them move in those bushes," James said as he pointed to the edge of the woods.

"I saw something move. But it looked more like a man, though," John said.

"It could have been another hunter. You don't think we are the only people that know this place hasn't been hunted in for over twenty-five years, do you?"

"I guess not," Jack answered. "But why doesn't he come over and say hello?"

"Maybe he's just shy. Besides I hope he doesn't come over here. The only thing I want to see this weekend is something I killed," James answered.

"I hate to tell you this, Dad, but I heard that this place is also open for motorcycle riders," Jack said.

"As long as they don't get in my way, I don't care. But if those noisy things scare away my game, I may hang their head in my trophy room."

Jack dropped a branch on the fire. His father had said it in a joking way, but there was no telling what his father would do if someone riding a motorcycle did spoil a shot, especially if he had been drinking.

"Let's get some food cooking. We brought some hot dogs for tonight, but tomorrow we'll eat what we kill," James said. He pulled the bottle of Bourbon from underneath the front seat of the car.

****

Thomas stepped back into the woods and stood behind a tree. He was certain that the young boy had seen him plainly. It didn't matter even if he had. He would take care of them tonight while they slept. He would have to be very careful with these people. They had guns, and they would not hesitate to use them.

Thomas knew it would not be as easy to kill these men as it had been the young couple.

Thomas walked deep into the woods and climbed to the top of a steep hill. He stood in front of a large clump of bushes. He slipped through a narrow opening between two of them and entered his home. It was a concrete bunker that he had equipped with running water by diverting a small stream that ran behind the bunker to run through a trench he had dug in the back of the bunker. It had taken him a year to break through the concrete floor to form his trench, but it had been worth the effort to him. On the hot days of summer he could have a cool drink of water without venturing outside into the steamy woods. In the winter time he could sit next to the fire and have plenty of water. Besides, time did not matter to him anymore than it did to the trees in the forest. His father had always told him that a man was like a tree and the animals in the woods; each of them had an allotted time to spend on this earth. When that time was up, then man, animal, and tree would return to the earth to be born again. Thomas had listened to everything his father had told him about life and the woods. Thomas had understood his father's words about life and death in the woods. He understood well that one animal must kill another to live. That was what Thomas had to do now. He had to kill all intruders so he could live his life in peace. The intruders would die and return to the earth. They might even come back as a tree in the forest, or a deer that could run as swift as the wind blew on a stormy night. The intruders would be much better off as a part of the forest. Thomas felt as if he were actually doing them a favor by killing them.

He had listened to his father and had remembered his words well. The things his father had taught him had allowed him to survive in the woods all these years without the modern conveniences. The bark of certain trees boiled in water had cured him of the winter chills that made him shiver even as he sat next to a roaring fire. The forest took care of its own. Thomas would do what he had to do to take care of the forest.

Thomas looked slowly around his sparsely furnished home. In one corner of the bunker was a pallet on the floor. It was made from a deer hide stuffed with pine straw. There was an extra hide that served as a blanket to cover him. The fur of a small raccoon stuffed with the feathers of many birds served as his pillow. In the other corner of the bunker was his dining area. An old stump the army men had dug up made a nice dining table. A smaller stump he used as a chair. He used several turtle shells ranging in size from large to small as his cooking pots and bowls. The bones of the animals he killed for food were his utensils. Thomas was proud of the fact that all the furnishings of his home had been provided by the forest. All except for one thing. That was the wire he used to build the cage in the far corner of his bunker. There was no need for him to venture out of his woods again for the rest of his life. His fireplace, which doubled as his stove, was located in the center of the large room. The smoke would drift upward and escape through an opening he had made in the roof of the bunker. He walked over to the stove and turned the meat he was cooking slowly over the low fire. Thomas liked the winter in the woods better than he did the summer because he could have meat everyday without hunting daily. He could kill a large animal, and the cold would prevent it from going bad overnight. Thomas only killed what he needed to survive. He pinched off a piece of the meat that was cooking over the fire and put it in his mouth. It had a tangy but sweet taste that could only be described as unique. He took another large bite of it. He decided that his job as keeper of the woods would have many rewards that he had not counted on.

The rumbling sound coming from the far corner of the bunker diverted his attention and he looked over in the direction from which the sound came.

"Be quiet!" he yelled.

The corner of the room fell silent again. He walked over to the wall where he had his extra meat hanging and pulled down a large piece. He looked it over closely. It would be enough to last for a while. He took the meat to the corner where the rumbling sound had emanated, opened the cage door and tossed the piece of meat into it.

"You don't need it cooked. You can eat it raw," he said as he watched the meat being devoured.

Thomas went back to the fire and ate his fill of the cooked meat. After he finished he let out a large belch and tossed the bone to the side. He took another piece of meat down from the wall and placed it over the fire. He would be hungry again later and it would be done by then.

He looked around the bunker before he left. His father had told him to always take a last look around your home before you leave because it may not be there when you returned. His father should know. The Army men had used a bulldozer and leveled his house while he was out hunting for food.

The rumbling from the cage in the corner of the room began again.

"You have had enough to eat for now. I'll be back later," he said as he slipped out the opening of the bunker and through the bushes.

CHAPTER 4

The Friday night before New Year's Eve finally came. Arthur was packed and ready to go camping with his son ,Sean, and J.P. Keller. As usual he was waiting for Sean to arrive to pick him up. Sean had told him he would be there at seven o'clock sharp. It was now nine-fifteen.

Arthur whiled away the time by riding his motorcycle up and down the long driveway. J.P. had been right when he told him that the art of riding a motorcycle would come back to him. Arthur would ride down the long driveway and cut between two Azalea bushes and back to the driveway again. The feel of the power beneath him made him remember the old days when he was a teenager and rode motorcycles all the time. Those days of riding for hours and feeling the wind rush through his hair and in his face had given Arthur a feeling of freedom and excitement in his life that he never knew he missed so much until this very moment. It also reminded him of the reason he had stopped riding. He had been broadsided by a little old lady who should have been driving a wheelchair instead of a car. The force had sent him sliding a hundred and fifty feet along the pavement. Amazingly enough, he had been able to get up and stand after he stopped sliding. He was checking his bike for damage when the old lady panicked and hit the gas pedal instead of her brakes and slammed into him again. Arthur was not as lucky the second time she hit him as he was the first time. He woke up in the hospital later with no memory of the past two weeks he had been in a coma. Arthur had not replaced that motorcycle. He knew his responsibilities as a father and provider for his family were much more important than his own pleasure.

As he waited for Sean he also remembered when Sean had bought his motorcycle a few weeks ago. Arthur had been consumed by a feeling of fear and impending doom. Sean had tried to comfort him and erase those feelings by explaining that he would not be riding a street motorcycle, he would be riding a trail bike. A car would not run over you in the woods. Sean had even laid out all the safety equipment he had bought for riding.

He had a sturdy helmet, a chest plate, knee pads, and riding boots that even the largest snake with fangs could not penetrate. Seeing all the safety equipment had alleviated most of Arthur's fears, but not all of them. He knew he would always worry about his kids no matter how old they were, or what they did.

Arthur stopped his motorcycle when he saw Elizabeth come out of the door and into the driveway.

"Sean's not here yet, I see," she said with a grin.

"No. But he's only a few hours late."

"You know Sean. He'll be here soon. Don't be so impatient. He said he had to get some last minute things for the trip. You and he and J.P. are going to have tonight and all weekend to have fun. A few hours is not going to make any difference."

"You're right," Arthur said as he leaned over and kissed her tenderly on the lips. "Are you sure you don't want to go with us?"

"No way. I'm going to stay here and play with the grandbabies. It's too cold for me anyway. I would rather sit home by the fire."

"We won't get to spend New Year's Eve together. It will be the first one in twenty-seven years we haven't spent together."

"We'll survive," Elizabeth replied. "It's more important to spend time with your son."

"You're right about that," Arthur said and kissed her on the lips again. "However, there will be other females there tomorrow when Sean's other friends come to ride."

"There are always women around Sean and J.P. You just make sure they are not around you," she said.

"Why would those young girls want to hang around an old guy like me?"

"You would be surprised what a young girl will do nowadays."

"You were a young girl once. You wouldn't do any of that until I married you."

"Times have changed. You just behave," Elizabeth teased.

Arthur flipped the switch on the handlebars and the engine died. He got off his motorcycle and put both his arms around Elizabeth and looked deeply into her eyes.

"As long as Sean is late, we may as well kill some time until he gets here," Arthur announced as he slipped his right hand beneath her blouse and caressed her left breast.

Before she could answer yes or no, the headlights lit up the driveway, and them. Arthur quickly removed his hand from beneath her blouse. Sean got out from the passenger side of the Suburban and started laughing.

"Didn't I teach you two better than to do the wild thing in the driveway?" he asked.

"Yes, you did. But I forgot," Arthur joked.

"What am I going to do with these old people, J.P.?" Sean asked him.

"Don't bring **me** into this," J.P. replied.

"I had to do something while I was waiting for you," Arthur said.

"You couldn't find anything else to do? It's a good thing we showed up when we did. You two would have been bumping uglies in another minute or two," Sean quickly added.

"Wait a minute. Who is the dad and who is the son around here?" J.P. asked.

"I'm beginning to wonder that myself."

Arthur decided not to answer Sean. If he did, Sean would come up with one of his other unique phrases and they would be standing in the driveway all night trading barbs. Arthur was proud of the relationship he had with his son. There were not many fathers who could joke with their sons the way he could with Sean. But they had their bad moments, too. Like the time Sean fell in with the wrong crowd when he was sixteen and started lying and doing some things he shouldn't have. Arthur had never worried so much and felt such heartache in his life. But Sean had seen the error of his ways and straightened himself out. Six months ago he had moved out on his own and rented a house. J.P. had moved in with him recently. The sound of J.P.'s voice pulled him from his thoughts.

"We had better get your bike loaded up, Mr. Billings," he said.

"Call me Arthur. It takes too long to say Mr. Billings."

"Okay, Arthur," Sean said. "Let's get that bike loaded up. We are wasting time."

Arthur sighed. It was just like Sean to show up late, then hurry everyone. He pushed his bike to the trailer behind the Suburban and lifted the front tire up on it as Sean pushed from behind. J.P. pulled the straps across the handlebars, tightened them up, and made sure the bike was secure.

"Let's go," J.P. said as he opened the driver's door to the Suburban and crawled behind the steering wheel.

Arthur ran over and kissed Elizabeth goodbye and got in the back seat. Sean sat in the front seat.

The Suburban was a large vehicle with a front seat that could seat three people comfortably. The back seat that Arthur sat in was the same size. The seat that was normally in the rear had been removed and Arthur saw the blankets lying in the empty space. He knew that area would be his sleeping quarters for the next couple of nights. He tried not to think about how his back was going to feel on Monday morning.

Elizabeth stood in the driveway and waved goodbye as they backed out. A cold chill suddenly came over her. She wanted to run after the vehicle and stop them. She fought the urge and convinced herself that it was just the cold night air that made her feel that way, and knowing that she would miss her husband.

"Be careful," she said softly as she watched them drive away.

****

James Foster sat by the campfire and finished the last drop of bourbon from the bottle and tossed it into the woods.

"I think it's about time we called it a night," he said to his two sons.

"Whatever you say, Dad," Jack answered.

"**That's what I said**. Are you arguing with me?"

"No, Sir," Jack answered quickly.

Jack knew better than to argue with his father, especially after he had been drinking.

"Then shut up and go to bed! And don't let that fire go out!" James shouted as he stumbled into his tent and crawled into his own sleeping bag. Within minutes he was sound asleep and snoring loudly.

"What makes him act that way?" John asked his brother.

"It's the booze. You know that as well as I do."

"I know, but what makes him drink? He's the greatest dad in the world when he isn't drinking. But he has been drinking a lot lately."

"He has been hitting the stuff a lot more than he usually does," John said.

"It must be the pressure of his job. I heard him tell Mom that business is slow and they may have to start laying people off."

"Dad shouldn't have to worry about that," John said. "He has been with that company for over twenty years."

"That's just it. He makes more money than anyone else. What better way is there for a company to save money than to get rid of the biggest wage earners?"

"But Dad has given his life to that company," John added.

"Do you think they care about that? No way. They will toss him out in less than a minute when the time comes," John stated.

"Who will they replace him with?"

"Probably some younger man that will work for a lot less money just to get some experience."

"It doesn't seem right to me," John said with sadness.

"Right and wrong doesn't have anything to do with it. That's the way it is," Jack said.

"It must really make Dad feel useless." John was starting to understand his dad more.

"You had better believe it. Why do you think he insisted on this hunting trip? He wants to prove to us, and himself, that he is just as good as he ever was, that he's not too old to do anything."

"At least I can understand it now," John said.

"I wish I could. I only hope that we don't run into any motorcycle riders tomorrow," Jack stated softly.

Thomas walked through his woods toward the camp of the man and two teenagers. They would surely be asleep by now, and he could figure out a way to deal with them. He topped the hill and was walking across the road when he saw the headlights coming toward him. He stepped back into the trees and watched it pass. It was a large vehicle whose engine clanked loudly and emitted a smell that almost turned his stomach. He remembered the smell from the bulldozers. It was diesel fuel. He let the vehicle pass before he stepped from the trees back onto the road again. He stood there trying to decide which ones to take care of first. He had no idea how many were in the large vehicle, or if they had weapons. He knew about the men in the camp. He remembered a bit of his father's advice. Stay with your first plan. He continued walking toward the camp of the man and two boys.

J.P. pulled the Suburban into a small clearing and stopped. He turned the headlights off but left the motor running.

They stepped outside and stood in the blackness of the night. There were no stars shining and there was no moon to cast any light on their campsite.

"I hate to ask a stupid question," J.P. finally said after a few moments had passed, "but did you bring a flashlight, Sean?"

"I bought one just for this trip. A good one, too. It has the big bulbs that could light up an area fifty feet around. It cost me thirty bucks," Sean answered.

"That's great. Go get it and we'll build a fire," J.P. said.

"Can't do that," Sean answered with a grin.

"*Why not?*"

"I forgot it at the house."

Arthur was surprised at J.P.'s reaction. He had almost expected him to get angry, or at least show some sign of exasperation. What he saw was totally different. J.P. and Sean

42

both began to laugh. Before long Arthur was laughing along with them. He understood now why Sean and J.P. were such good friends. They both accepted the other the way they were. One did not try to change the other. A friendship like that was rare in today's world where most people treated friends lightly. Arthur had a friend like that, too. The best man in his wedding, Phillip Oliver. They had been friends since high school, and still were. He was glad that Sean had the same type of friendship with J.P.

"I hate to interrupt this male bonding experience," Arthur said, "but I am freezing."

"So am I," J.P. said as he got into the Suburban and turned on the headlights so they could see their surroundings. "We can break off some of those low hanging limbs on those trees and build a fire."

Within minutes they had a roaring fire going and sat around it telling stories and jokes. Arthur listened intently as J.P. talked of his childhood and all the different types of motorcycles he had when he was growing up. Arthur listened, not out of necessity, but out of interest. J.P. was an extremely intelligent person, but did not flaunt it. As he listened, Arthur wondered if there was anything about motorcycles or car engines that J.P. did not know.

Arthur did notice a few peculiarities that J.P. did have, however. For instance, when Arthur lit a cigarette and J.P. was about to smoke one, he would take the lighter from his hand and light it himself. It was as if it was not manly to let another man light his cigarette. Another one was opening doors for him. When they had stopped on the road to fill up and were heading into the restaurant, Arthur had instinctively opened the door and told J.P. to go in first. J.P. had politely refused and gone into the restaurant last.

Arthur didn't let those things bother him. If they were the only oddities J.P. had, they would get along fine. Away from everyone else, J.P. opened up and really talked about many things.

After they had talked for a while and swapped stories about the wild oats they had sown in their youth, it was time to go to sleep. They crawled into the Suburban. Sean and Arthur got on the floor in the rear and J.P. covered up with a blanket on the back seat. That was another of his little quirks. J.P. was not about to sleep next to a man, even if it was his best friend.

J.P. leaned over the seat and smiled.

"Before I turn off the light I would like to go over a couple of the rules of sleeping in close quarters like this."

"J.P.'s got a rule for **everything**," Sean whispered.

"As I was saying," J.P. continued. "Rule number one, no farting in the Suburban."

"Is that it? You said a couple of rules."

"That's the other rule, too."

"I wish you had told me that before I ate those two bean burritos. Don't worry, I'll hold it until morning," Sean said as he covered his head with the blanket.

"Everybody set?" J.P. asked as he turned out the overhead light in the Suburban.

"What if I had said no?" Sean asked.

"Too late now. One more thing I forgot to mention. I locked that back door from the outside. If one of you has to get up in the middle of the night, you'll have to crawl over me. Please wake me up first. I don't want any feet on my balls," J.P. instructed.

Arthur lay on the floorboard and stared up at the black sky. The only light around them was from the flickering flames of the slowly dying fire. He could hear Sean's breathing next to him as it became deeper and deeper. He would be asleep soon. Arthur could not tell if J.P. was asleep or not. He did know one thing. He was glad that J.P. had come with them. He was glad that he had the type of relationship with Sean that he did. Sean was a good son. Sure, Sean got on his nerves once in a while by being late and putting things off until the last minute and then rushing to get everything done. But that was the way Sean did things. It still irritated Arthur a lot when Sean did those things. He had decided long ago to accept the irritations and to accept Sean. Arthur knew there was no amount of preaching or complaining that was going to change the way Sean was. Sean was an extremely good-hearted person and had many friends. Arthur

44

liked the majority of them, and they liked him. Mark Helms was one of the ones that Arthur liked a lot. Mark had even lived with them for a while before Sean moved out on his own. He had stayed for two weeks until he could get his utilities turned back on. Mark was not any trouble at all while he lived in their house. In fact, it was a sad day for Arthur when Mark got back on his feet financially and moved out. Arthur missed talking to him and having someone to drink coffee with at five-thirty in the morning. Sean had many other friends, too, and most of them would be here tomorrow. But Mark and J.P. were Arthur's favorites.

Arthur stared at the sky. The fire was almost out now, and there were only a few intermittent sparks that passed by the window. His eyes grew heavy as he thought of all the joy he had experienced through the years of being a husband and a father. Arthur Billings considered himself a lucky man. Not only did he have Sean, but Sean's friends were almost like his sons, too. Mark even called him Dad.

Arthur had a great wife, too. Elizabeth had just turned seventeen when they were married twenty-five years ago. Arthur knew that if he had not married her so young, before she developed into the beautiful woman she became, he would not have had a chance with her. She would have been able to have her pick of any man she wanted. Yes, he considered himself a **very lucky man**.

The steady rhythm of Sean's breathing told Arthur that Sean was sleeping peacefully. A low snort from the seat above him told him that J.P. was sound asleep, too. These two boys worked so hard. J.P. was a mechanic, and Sean was part owner in Elizabeth's Beauty Salon. They played hard, too. They knew how to enjoy life to the fullest and not let the setbacks in life get them discouraged. They took the good with the bad and took it all in stride.

Arthur did not fight the sleep as it slowly overtook him. He closed his eyes and thought about tomorrow. It was going to be a great day. He was going to feel the wind in his soul again. He was going to feel the power beneath him once more. He might even be able to recapture the thrill of his youth.

Tomorrow was going to be a truly unforgettable day.

****

Thomas stood ten feet from the two tents. He could feel the heat of the roaring fire on his face and it angered him. These idiots had not dug up the area around the fire to prevent it from spreading. If it had not rained a couple of days ago and the ground had not been still wet, the fire would have surely spread to the trees and beyond. It might even have burned down the entire forest. It angered him even more that they had gone to sleep and had not even considered that possibility. He was going to enjoy getting rid of these interlopers even more than he had thought he would in the beginning.

The longer he stood there, the more intense his anger grew. He raised his stick and went toward the tent where the man was sleeping. He would probably be the most dangerous of the three.

As he approached the tent, Thomas held his stick as high as he could over his head. His heart pounded and his pulse raced as each step took him nearer to the one who had violated his peace. Thomas stood over the tent and brought the stick crashing down onto the area where he thought the man was lying. The tent collapsed as Thomas watched for any sign of movement.

"What the Hell are you doing?" Jack yelled from the other tent.

Before he could turn toward the youth, he heard the sound of a gunshot and felt the wind from the bullet pass by his head. As he ran into the woods, he heard the sound of several more gunshots from behind him. Exhausted and out of breath, he finally reached the safety of the woods and stood behind a huge pine tree and watched the confusion in the camp.

"Who the hell was that?" James Foster asked as he slowly lowered his rifle.

"I don't know. I couldn't get a good look at him," Jack answered.

"I did," John said. "It was the same man we saw standing at the edge of the woods earlier when we first arrived."

"It doesn't matter who it was anyway," James said. "What the Hell was he trying to do?"

Jack went to his father's tent and looked down at the tear the stick had made in it.

"It looks to me like he was trying to kill you."

"**Why** would he do that?"

"I don't know, but one thing is for certain, he wasn't trying to make friends with you," Jack stated.

"This is no time for smart aleck remarks. If I hadn't been taking a leak behind the car, that bastard would have killed me," James said.

"Do you <u>always</u> take your rifle when you take a leak,Dad?"

"Did you ever hear of rattlesnakes?" James asked with an angry tone to his voice.

"Did you hit him, Dad?" John asked. He wished that Jack would shut up and not make this situation any worse than it was by making his father angry.

"I don't think so. It was too dark to get a good shot at him."

"And you had too much to drink," Jack accused.

"If you've got something to say boy, spit it out," James ordered.

"All right, I will. You are the best shot I have ever seen. When you're sober, that is. Do you see what your drinking has caused? It could have been me or John with our head crushed in. If we don't get out of here right now, it still might be."

"Well, you don't have your head crushed, and you won't. One of us is going to stand guard the rest of the night. If that lunatic comes back, we'll take care of him for good," James said with certainty.

"Why can't we just get out of here now?" Jack asked.

"Because **no one** is going to run me off ever again. They did it at the office yesterday, and by God, I won't be run away from here."

"I'm sorry, Dad. I didn't know."

"It's no big deal. There are a lot of companies out there that will be begging me to come to work for them as soon as I let them know I'm available."

"I know that, Dad, but that doesn't have anything to do with

47

right now. It makes no sense for us to stay here and risk our lives," Jack pleaded.

James took two large steps and was standing next to Jack. He grabbed him by the collar of his shirt and put his face next to his.

Jack smelled the stale bourbon on his father's breath and turned his head away.

"Look at me, boy!" he said as he shook him.

Jack took a deep breath and looked at his father.

"It has everything to do with now. In fact, I couldn't have planned it better if I had tried. I brought you boys out here this weekend to teach you a few of the facts of life that I neglected to before. One of them is to never let anyone shit on you. This world is a rough place and I won't always be around to protect you. The other thing I wanted to teach you was to never let anyone run you off, no matter who they are."

"I still think we should leave and call the police," Jack said.

"And what would we tell them? We could tell them that we are helpless and need them to wipe our noses. I'll never admit that. The cops are the last people I want to see anyway."

Jack knew it was useless to argue with his father. It had never worked before. He saw no reason it should now. He remained silent until James released his grip on him and walked away and stared into the woods in the direction the man had gone.

"What are we going to do then?" he asked after a couple of minutes had passed.

His father turned around and Jack could see his expression by the firelight. It was an expression he had never seen on his father's face before. It bore a resemblance to a mad scientist he had seen on one of the old black and white horror movies. It was a sinister expression.

"We came up here to hunt, boy, didn't we? Well, that is exactly what we are going to do. We are going to hunt that son-of-a-bitch that tried to beat my brains out. It will be a lot more interesting than hunting deer anyway. A deer can't carry a stick. That guy is probably hauling ass out of these woods right now, but we'll find him as soon as it gets daylight. We'll hunt him down like a dog, then I'll put a bullet in his head. I'll teach him not to try and kill me."

Jack felt a cold chill race up and down his spine as his father spoke. There was something wrong. In the past, his father had always been so protective of him and his brother that he bordered on being ridiculous. He wouldn't even let them play pool at the local game room because he suspected that they would be exposed to drug dealers. Now, his father was willing to let them stay overnight in the woods where a madman who had just tried to kill him was lurking.

Jack wondered if the stress of losing his job had made his father cross the line that separated the sane from the insane. He also wondered who posed the bigger threat, the madman in the woods or his father.

CHAPTER 5

Thomas stood next to the tree and listened as the man spoke. "What an idiot," he said to himself. The man had revealed his plan loudly and plainly for him to hear. The man was foolish for thinking that he had run away. Thomas thought he was foolish, but in a strange way he admired the man for his principles. Thomas thought that he and the man in the tent were a lot alike. The man did not want to be run away from his job, and Thomas did not want to be run out of his woods. The man had allowed them to run him away from his job. That was where the man and he were different. He would not be run out of his woods by anyone, no matter who it was.

For the first time in his life, Thomas felt a twinge of regret that he would have to kill the man. He knew it would not bother him to kill the two boys. The man would make a good companion. Thomas hated to admit it, but once in a while, and it was not very often, but every now and then he felt lonely to talk to someone. He especially wanted to talk to someone besides the occupant of the cage in his bunker.

Thomas watched the campsite as the man barked his orders to his sons. He saw them set up a wire around the perimeter to warn them if anyone came near the tents.

Thomas almost laughed at their working so hard at what was clearly a waste of time. He would not go back to the camp tonight. The man was wrong when he said that Thomas was running away. The man was wrong about something else, too. Thomas rubbed his arm and felt the blood flowing from the wound. The man was wrong when he said that he had missed him when he shot at him.

Thomas walked through the woods and headed for his bunker. On the way he stopped at the other campsite. These people were smarter. They were sleeping in a locked vehicle. He had no way of knowing how many there were, or if they had guns. He would have to catch them tomorrow. That would not be hard to do. They would crawl on their noisy motorcycles and separate as they tore through the woods killing every small plant in their path. The smoke from their exhausts would smell up his forest and make some of the smaller animals sick. He would truly enjoy ridding his woods of these people, no matter how many there were of them. They would be easy to get, too. All he would have to do is get them one at a time as they drove past him. And he would make sure they drove past him, at least once. If Thomas had his way, the first time they passed him would be their last.

A small twinge of pain went through his arm and he grabbed it. The bleeding had started again, so he headed for his bunker quickly.

****

Arthur opened his eyes and it took a moment for him to realize where he was. Sean had pulled the blanket off of him, and he was cold. He rose up and looked over the seat at J.P. J.P. was just as sound asleep as Sean was. He wiped the sleep from his eyes and looked out the window. The sun was still not up, but it was light enough for him to see the frost covered ground.

He crawled over the seat and over J.P. Then he opened the side door and stepped out. Arthur immediately felt the blast of cold air hit him in the face. His hands began to shake instantly in spite of the cotton gloves he wore. He gathered a few branches and began to make a fire. The branches were still damp, so he did what they had done the night before. He poured some gasoline from the can on the trailer on the wood and lit it. He had a roaring blaze going in a matter of seconds. He gathered more wood and threw it on the fire. For a while he didn't think he was ever going to warm up. After standing near the fire for several minutes, he finally felt the warmth come over him. Then something else came over him. It was a feeling, a feeling of being watched. He had concentrated so much on getting the fire built, that he had not even looked around him. Now that he was warm, the feeling dominated his very being. He turned his head slowly and looked around him. He was surrounded by a whole herd of cows. They were inching closer toward him as he stood there staring at them.

"Good morning, Mr. Billings, I mean Arthur," J.P. said as he walked over to the fire.

"Morning, Arthur," Sean said as he followed closely behind J.P.

"Good morning, guys, we have company," Arthur said as he pointed to the cows around them.

Sean and J.P. looked at the cows. J.P. pulled a clump of grass and walked slowly toward a big brown one.

"You want some breakfast?" he asked as he held the grass in front of him.

A big, white bull with one horn that pointed straight down and another horn that stood straight up began to stamp his feet and snort as J.P. got nearer to the cow.

"I think you're messing with his woman, J.P." Sean said.

J.P. dropped the grass and returned to the fire. The bull then calmed down but did not take his eyes off of J.P.

"What got him in such a bad mood?" J.P. asked.

"Maybe he's horny," Sean said.

Arthur and J.P. rolled their eyes at Sean.

"That was pretty corny,Sean, " Arthur said.

"It wasn't bad for this early in the morning," Sean replied.

The bull began to snort and stamp his feet again. He reared straight up and ran toward them. They moved to the other side of the fire and the bull ran past them and chased the big brown cow away from the rest of the herd. He went behind the cow and mounted her.

"I **told you** he was horny," Sean laughed. "He got mad at J.P. for messing with his nookie."

"He may be horny, but I'm hungry," J.P. said.

"And I need a cup of coffee," Arthur added.

"I'm hungry, too," Sean said. "There's a small cafe a few miles from the main road. I heard they have biscuits there that are the size of hubcaps."

"When is everyone else going to get here?" Arthur asked.

"Who knows! They are always late," Sean said.

"You should talk," Arthur mumbled as he put out the fire.

They got back in the Suburban and headed for the cafe.

****

Thomas sat in his bunker dressing his wound. It was not serious at all. The bullet had just grazed his arm. He should have known when there was not much pain that it wasn't bad. He knew he always bled freely from even the slightest scratch. He applied a mixture of mud and a few of the herbs he kept around the bunker to his arm. It immediately soothed the minor pain and stopped the bleeding.

The rattling in the cage irritated Thomas more than the wound. He got up and walked over to the cage and kicked it. The occupant scurried toward the far corner of the cage.

"**What's your problem this morning**?" he shouted.

The only sound that came from the cage was a low growl.

"Are **you** hungry again?"

Thomas looked down and saw the large bone from the piece of meat he had thrown into the cage the night before.

"You ate all that already? You are more trouble than you are worth," he said as he walked over and pulled another large piece of meat down from the rack.

Thomas went back to the cage and held the meat in front of the cage door as he teased the occupant with it.

"You want some more?" he asked as the occupant came to the door and tried to get the meat.

Thomas kicked the door and the occupant scurried back to the corner again.

"I'm going to be gone most of the day. I guess I had better feed you now. I don't want you gnawing off your foot," Thomas said as he opened the door and threw in the meat that he had set aside.

Thomas watched as the occupant of the cage grabbed the meat, tore it to shreds, and almost swallowed it without chewing.

"You are getting pretty big. I'm going to have to build you a bigger cage before long. If I could trust you to behave yourself, I wouldn't have to keep you locked up all the time," he sneered.

Thomas looked for a reaction from the occupant. There was none. All he heard was the low growling sound that came from deep within the occupant's throat as it devoured the meat.

"I wish I could trust you not to bite me again, like you did the last time I tried to let you out of that cage," Thomas said as he looked at the long, jagged scar that ran from his elbow to his wrist. Thomas was injured when he jerked his arm from the mouth of the occupant of the cage.

"I guess you are not ready for freedom yet. Well, the time will come sooner or later. Right now I have to go and take care of some trespassers. There are three of them camped in the north meadow, and there are some more camped about a mile from there. I don't know how many there are in that second car, but I'll find out. There are three motorcycles on that trailer, so I know there are at least three of them. But there may be more, some of them may be riding double. It doesn't matter anyway. No matter how many of them there are, they are all going to die before the sun goes down tonight. That's a promise. I think I'll take care of them first. They should be up and ready to ride by the time I get to them."

Thomas expected no answer from the occupant of the cage, and he was not disappointed when he didn't get one. He left the bunker and climbed down the hill and went through the woods to the camp of the motorcycle riders. The big vehicle was gone. This did disappoint him. He knew they would be back. These city people probably went into town to get breakfast. They didn't know how to survive in the woods. He almost wished that he could take days to kill them. That way he could enjoy watching them try to live off the land. He could watch them slowly starve to death. He pushed that thought from his mind quickly. They were trespassers, and they had to die. The sooner the better. He headed for the other camp. He knew they would be there. They would be up and ready to come hunting for him.

A low chuckle escaped from his throat. The hunters were about to become the hunted.

****

"Wake up! Get your asses up and ready to go!" James shouted at the two boys.

John and Jack woke up and exited their tent quickly. James handed them their rifles.

"Load up and bring some extra bullets," he ordered.

The boys did not question their father. They knew it would not do any good.

"I packed the knapsack with some food. There's no telling how long it will take us to find him. But we won't come back until we do."

The boys watched their father as he went back to the car and pulled another full bottle of bourbon from beneath the seat. He took a long drink from it and put it in the knapsack. Then he put the knapsack on his back and started walking into the woods.

"What are we going to do?" John asked. He was only fourteen and more scared than he had ever been in his life. He wished he could be more like Jack. Jack was sixteen and as strong as an ox. John always looked up to Jack. He could handle any situation with calmness. He was also envious of Jack. His father was always bragging to his few friends how good an athlete Jack was. He never said anything about his being on the Honor Roll ever since the third grade.

"Follow him I guess," Jack said. "Have you got your inhaler?"

John suffered from asthma, and as a result, was thin and sickly looking. He was a constant source of worry for Jack.

"Yes, I have it."

"Good, let's go."

They had to run to catch up with their father since he was walking so fast. They caught up with him just as he reached the edge of the woods.

"Spread out," James said. "John, you go twenty feet to my left. Jack, you go twenty feet to my right. If you see him, don't hesitate. Shoot to kill."

Jack and John looked at each other and followed their father's instructions. John ran his fingers over the wooden stock of his rifle. He had never killed anything in his life. His father had constantly reminded him of that fact every time they returned from a hunting trip. He secretly wished that he would spot the man first. If he did, he would do his best to pull the trigger and kill the man. He had no doubt that the memory would haunt his dreams and his waking hours for the rest of his life. But it would be worth it if he could hear his father brag to his friends how his youngest son, John, the son that had been ill most of his life, the son who couldn't play football or baseball like his brother did, had killed the man who tried to kill him. It would be worth every bit of sleep he lost for the rest of his life if he could hear his father brag on him just one time.

John slipped the safety off the rifle and slid a bullet into the chamber. He wiped the sweat from his hands onto his shirt. He narrowed his eyes into small slits and scanned every inch of the woods in front of him. He was ready to kill the man the instant he saw him. He was ready to make his father proud of him.

CHAPTER 6

Arthur, Sean, and J.P. sat at the table in the far corner of the cafe. The dining room was large and could easily hold over a hundred people. Arthur guessed that before the military base closed, this place was packed every day. Now there were only three people besides them in the cafe.

A waitress with the bottom row of her teeth missing and the top row filled with black ones brought over three cups of coffee and set them down on the table.

"I'll have a Dr. Pepper," Sean said.

"Me, too," J.P. agreed.

"You mean you don't want any coffee?" she asked.

"No, thank you," Sean answered.

"I'll have to pour it back into the pot," she whined.

"Don't worry about it," Arthur interrupted. "I'll drink all three cups. Just bring them each a Dr. Pepper."

"If that's what you want, all right. I never heard of anyone drinking Dr. Pepper instead of coffee with their breakfast."

"I heard coffee rots your teeth," Sean mumbled under his breath.

Arthur kicked Sean lightly on his leg under the table. "Be nice," he whispered.

They watched the waitress walk slowly back across the large dining room. She was fat and her rear end hung behind her and made her look like she was wearing a diaper.

"I'll bet there are a lot of things she hasn't heard of," Sean said. "She probably was born here and hasn't been anywhere else since that day."

"Not everyone is as well traveled as you are," J.P. joked.

Arthur drank all three cups of coffee while they waited for the waitress to bring the Dr. Peppers and a menu.

Twenty minutes passed before Arthur got up and went behind the counter and poured himself another cup of coffee.

"That's my job," the waitress said as he sat back down.

"I'm sorry. I didn't see you anywhere," Arthur answered.

"Just don't let it happen **again**," she said as she turned to walk away.

"Excuse me ma'am," J.P. said, "but we still don't have our Dr. Peppers."

"I thought you wanted them with your breakfast."

"We could drink one now, and another one with our breakfast."

"If that's what you want. I still never heard of such a thing though. I'll go get them," the waitress announced.

"Excuse me again, Ma'am, but we don't have a menu."

"The breakfast menu is on the wall, over there," she said as she pointed to a chalkboard.

They read the handwritten menu.

"Pancakes, eggs, bacon."

"What else do you have? Do you offer any other items?" J.P. asked.

"Do you see anything else written on that board?" she asked him.

"No."

"**Then that's all we have**," the waitress replied with impatience.

Sean studied the chalkboard seriously for a full minute.

"I think I'll have the pancakes, eggs, and bacon," he said in his most serious voice.

"Me, too," Arthur said.

"I guess I'll have what they are having," J.P. added. "But don't bring me any eggs. I don't eat eggs."

"I still have to charge you for them," the waitress told him.

"That's all right."

The waitress looked at Sean.

"How do you want your eggs?"

"Over medium, with the white done, and the yellow runny."

"And you?" she asked as she shifted her gaze to Arthur.

"The same way."

"And how do you want yours?" she asked J.P..

"I **don't want** any eggs," J.P. impatiently replied.

"Oh, yes. I forgot," she said.

They did their best not to burst out with laughter as the

waitress walked behind the counter and went through a swinging door.

"Where do they find these people?" J.P. finally asked.

"You have to realize how hard it is to find good help in the middle of nowhere," Arthur said. "The only thing this area had going for it was the money from the soldiers on the base. Now that they are gone, so is most of their business. They probably give her room and board to work here. Judging from the amount of customers here, the owner sure couldn't afford to pay her."

"Why don't they just lock the door and leave?" Sean asked.

"More than likely, the owner has lived in this area all his life. This is his home. As long as he can barely survive, he'll hold on. Maybe now that the camp has been reopened to the public, business will pick up."

"He had better hire another waitress," J.P. said.

"I don't know about that," Sean said. "She's kind of sexy with those teeth missing."

This time they could not control the urge to laugh out loud. Their laughter filled the cafe and echoed around the almost empty room.

One of the men sitting at the table on the end got up and walked over to their table. He wore a pair of blue overalls with one strap hanging loosely. He also wore a green cap with "John Deere" emblazoned on the front of it. The corners of his mouth were brown from the tobacco he was chewing.

"Y'all aren't from around here, are you?" he asked.

"No. We just came up here to ride at Camp Leder," Arthur answered.

"Them there your motorcycles on that trailer out there?" he asked as he pointed out the window.

"Yes," Arthur answered as his laughter subsided.

"Y'all going to ride them in those woods?" he questioned.

"That's the plan," Arthur said.

"I don't know as I reckon that's such a good idea."

"Why is that?" Arthur asked.

"Don't rightly know. They got a lot of snakes in those woods. Rattlesnakes, big ones too," the man replied.

"We've seen snakes before. We've even had to kill a few."

"They got some wild cows out there," the man added.

"I know. We met some of them this morning," Arthur stated.

"It's mighty cold out there. That wind will cut through you like a knife," the man warned.

"Is there anything else that you can tell us about those woods?" Arthur asked with defiance in his voice. "Are you telling us that we shouldn't ride in those woods?"

"I ain't telling you nothing. Ain't none of my business what you do. I'm just trying to warn you."

"Warn us about what? Snakes, cows, the cold?"

"There's something else in those woods, something strange," the man said.

"What do you mean by that?"

"I can't explain it. I heard stories," he added with hesitancy in his voice.

"What kind of stories?"

"Stories those soldier boys used to tell. They said they had the feeling that they were always being watched. No matter where they went in those woods, they had that feeling."

"They were probably smoking some wacky-tobaccy," Sean joked.

"You can laugh if you want to, but there **is** something strange in those woods. People tell me about seeing headlights going down that main road at night and never seeing them come out again," he continued.

"Maybe they spent the night and left the next morning," J.P. said.

"Maybe so. All I know is I've lived in this area for over sixty years. I have never set one foot in those woods, and I don't reckon I ever will."

"Thanks for the warning," Arthur said.

"Get out of the way," the waitress told the man as she set the plates on the table.

The man nodded and returned to his table.

They looked at the plates the waitress had placed on the table in front of them. All three plates contained eggs that were scrambled.

"Excuse me, miss, but we wanted our eggs over medium, and he didn't want any eggs," Sean said.

"Don't worry about it, Sean," J.P. interrupted. "We're burning daylight. Let's just eat and get out of here."

They quickly dug into their food with a ravenous hunger that had been building since they had first awakened. But after two bites, J.P. put his fork down.

"What's the matter?" Arthur asked him.

"There's something in those pancakes that don't belong there."

"Mine taste kind of funny, too," Sean said.

"Why don't we grab a few candy bars at that little store we passed on the way here?" Arthur suggested.

"Sounds good to me," Sean and J.P. agreed in unison. Sean signalled to the waitress for the ticket and she came over and held it out to him. As he reached for it, she pulled it away, held it out and pulled it away again. The third time she held it out, she pulled it away and handed it to Arthur.

"I'll get it," Sean said. "The meals are a part of the Christmas present."

"Are you sure?"

"Let the boy pay for it," the waitress said.

Then she leaned over and whispered in J.P.'s ear. "If you didn't like the food, don't say anything to anybody. You'll get me in trouble."

"What was that all about?" Arthur asked as the waitress walked away from the table.

"I don't know," J.P. answered, "and I don't care. Let's just get out of here."

As they left the cafe after Sean paid the ticket, they passed the old man who had come over to their table.

"Be careful in those woods," he said.

"We will. We appreciate your warning."

"And may God have mercy on you," the man said grimly.

They rode back to their campsite in an unnatural silence. Arthur tried to forget the man's words of warning, but he couldn't. He also could not shake the uneasy feeling that was growing stronger with each mile that brought them closer to the woods.

****

James, Jack, and John Foster trudged through the woods with one thing on their minds. They wanted to find the man who had invaded their camp the night before, and two of them wanted to find the man and kill him. They were oblivious to the cold morning air. Their eyes searched every part of the ground in front of and to the side of them for any sign of the direction the man from the night before had taken.

Jack was nervous. He was usually unshakable in times of emergency. He always stayed calm when others would panic. This was different though. His father was obsessed with finding the man. That, he could understand. His father was like that. The thing he couldn't understand was his younger brother, John. He seemed to be just as obsessed as his father was, maybe even more so.

Jack looked over in the direction of his father. He had stopped and had taken a large drink from the bottle. It was already half empty. If his father kept drinking like that, he would not be able to see the man if he bumped into him.

Jack looked past his father at John. He was acting like a great white hunter stalking a beast in the jungle. His eyes were fixed on the ground in front of him. His finger was dangerously close to the trigger of his rifle. The expression on his brother's face scared Jack. It was the same one his father wore.

He was staring at them so intently that he almost tripped over a dead tree that was lying in his path.

"I found something!" John yelled.

"What is it?" James asked.

"I think it's blood!"

James and Jack ran over to the spot where John was pointing.

"It is blood!" James said with excitement in his voice. "I hit him last night."

"It could be the blood of an animal," Jack said.

"Bullshit!" John snapped. "If Dad said he hit him, he hit him."

"That's the way to tell him, boy. John, you keep this up and you might turn out all right yet."

"I wasn't saying you didn't hit him, Dad. I just meant we can't be sure," Jack answered.

"Well, you'll be sure when we find him lying in the woods up ahead somewhere. He'll either be dead or bleeding to death."

"I still think we ought to let the police handle this," Jack argued.

"I told you I don't want to be around any police. If a man can't protect himself and his family, he's got no business living. And neither does his family."

"Whatever you say, Dad. But we should take it slow. He may not be hurt that bad."

"Are you serious?" James asked. "Look at the size of those blood drops. There are probably a hundred more behind us that we missed."

"I didn't miss any, Dad," John said quickly.

"I didn't mean you did, John. You did good finding these. I only meant that some pine needles could have fallen over some other signs of blood."

"I'll keep looking real good, Dad."

"I know you will, boy. I'm proud of you. Maybe if your brother was not so busy seeing how many drinks I've been taking from this bottle, he could have found some blood drops, too."

"I've been looking, Dad. But I'm also worried about John. This excitement is not good for his asthma."

"You let me worry about John. You just keep your damn eyes on the ground in front of you!"

"Yes, sir."

"I'm glad we got that settled. Let's spread out in this area, but close the gap between us," James ordered as he took another long drink from the bottle and returned it to the knapsack.

They walked for another hundred yards before they found another few drops of blood. Jack found them this time. He called his father and John over and showed them the drops.

"Now we're getting somewhere," James said. "He can't be very far from here."

"Doesn't it seem odd to you, Dad?" Jack asked.

"What are you talking about?"

"The trail is leading away from the road. If the man was wounded that badly, wouldn't he head for the road?" Jack questioned his father.

"*Why would he do that?*"

"Because it would be the fastest way to get help."

"He would have had to pass our camp to get back to the road."

"Not necessarily. There are at least a hundred places he could have cut through the woods to reach the road. Yet, the trail is leading to higher ground and away from the road," Jack responded.

"What are you getting at?"

"I think he left those blood drops for us to find. I think he's leading us right where he wants us to be, Dad," Jack added.

James shook his head in disgusted surprise. "Let me see if I have this straight," he said. "You are trying to tell me that a man that is stupid enough to charge into a camp occupied by three people with guns and try to bash my brains out with a big stick is clever enough to plant blood drops on the trail so we will follow them into his trap. Is that what you are trying to tell me?"

"All I'm saying is that if he was hurt that badly, he would be trying to get help," Jack argued.

"Well let's just suppose, for the moment, that he is hurt as bad as I think he is. Did you ever think **he may be hiding** from the police? That may be the reason he's in these woods in the first place. If he is wanted by the police, he wouldn't be dumb enough to go to a hospital. They are required to report all gunshot wounds to the authorities."

"I think he would rather be in jail than dead," Jack answered.

"That's where you are wrong, Son. There are many men in this world that would rather be dead than in jail. I am one of them."

Jack noticed the change in his father's eyes. There was something terribly wrong. It was not just his obsession with finding this man. There was something much deeper than that bothering his father. He only prayed he could find out what it was before they all were killed.

"What do you think, John?" James asked his other son.

"I think the answer is simple. The man panicked when you shot him. He ran into the woods and got lost. Look at the place where we found that other blood in relation to this one. He seems to be wandering toward the high ground because he has lost his sense of direction. It was dark out here last night. The man probably thought he was going toward the road, but got mixed up in the dark and came this way instead."

"That makes a lot of sense to me," James agreed.

"I also think we are wasting valuable time," John added. "If we don't find him soon, he'll bleed to death."

"That would be a real pity," James said.

"It sure would. I wanted to be the one to finish him off," John announced.

"That's my boy!! Let's go get him!"

Jack followed them as they went through the woods following several drops of blood they found every forty or fifty feet. He was worried even more by John's remarks now than he was before. At least he had figured out what was going on inside John's mind. He was starving for positive recognition from their father. He wanted and needed that recognition so badly that he would do anything to get it, including kill.

The man and his two sons were watching the ground ahead of them so intensely that they did not bother to look behind them. If they had turned around quickly enough, they might have caught a glimpse of the tall, shadowy figure that followed behind them, the figure that walked silently through the forest and was not in the hurry that they were. For Thomas knew where they were going. And Thomas also planned that they would not be coming back.

CHAPTER 7

Arthur, Sean, and J.P. unloaded their motorcycles from the trailer.

Arthur watched as Sean and J.P. put on their chest plates, heavy riding gloves, and steel toed riding boots. He wore a pair of Wal-Mart black dress boots.

"What about me? I don't have a chest plate, and these boots are not going to stop a snake from biting me," Arthur joked.

"Sorry, Dad. I didn't have any money left after I bought the motorcycle and the parts to fix it up. We did get you a helmet, though," Sean said.

"Don't worry about it," J.P. said. "You won't be going through some of the places we will. Not today anyway. You need to spend the day getting used to riding again."

"I'll go along with that. I just want to take it slow and easy."

"You can take it easy, but you won't be taking it slow," Sean laughed.

"Besides, Sean said he was going to get you a pair of riding boots for Father's Day," J.P. said.

"Thanks a lot, J.P."

"Oops! Forget I said that."

J.P. handed an old red helmet to Arthur, and he slipped it over his head. It was too big and fell over his eyes.

"Don't worry about that, Dad. We figured it would be too big. That's why we brought this." Sean handed Arthur a blue dish towel.

"What am I supposed to do with this?" Arthur asked.

"Fold it up and put it in the top of the helmet. It'll fit fine then," Sean answered quickly.

Arthur had his doubts, but he folded the towel and put it in the helmet. Then he tried the helmet on again. It fit almost perfectly.

"I'll never doubt you again," Arthur said meekly.

"Yes, you will," Sean grinned.

J.P. waited until they had finished their friendly joking before he spoke. "Please excuse me, gentlemen. It's time to go over the rules."

"*More rules*," Sean said as he rolled his eyes.

He noticed the seriousness in J.P.'s expression and leaned against his bike. J.P. didn't get serious very often, but when he did, it was important.

"Now that I have your attention, I will continue. From what I have heard, these trails are tricky and extremely dangerous. It's not hard to get lost, either. So we need to try and always keep within sight of each other. There are also a lot of snakes in these woods. They probably won't be out in the open because it's so cold, but we could always fall on one of them. That might make them mad." J.P. warned.

"I know it would me," Sean interrupted.

J.P. waited to make sure Sean was finished with his jokes. After a long pause, he decided he was.

"As I was saying, we need to be extra careful until we learn these trails. Now, Mr. Billings ...."

"Call me Arthur."

"Arthur, if you go through any mud, don't be surprised if you do a lot of sliding. You have street tires on your bike instead of mud tires. They hold the mud in the treads and it's hard to get traction with the mud on them. As you ride, the mud will fly off, and you can get traction again."

Arthur stood and listened as J.P. and Sean gave him a crash course in dirt bike riding. They told him so many things that after a while all of their instructions seemed to flow together and collect into a large mass of what to do and what not to do, and when not to do it.

Arthur knew that he would learn most of the things they were telling him not to do when he did them. After a while, the lesson was over.

"Are we ready to ride and have fun?" J.P. asked.

No one needed to answer that question. Sean kicked the crank on his bike, and the engine roared. Arthur did the same. Although his bike was over twenty years old, J.P. had done such a good job rebuilding the engine, it started on the first try just as Sean's had.

Sean and Arthur watched as J.P. stood on the side of his bike. His bike was a Honda 500cc and stood almost as tall as he was. He had to put his boot high into the air for his foot to reach the crank. He jumped up and brought his full weight down on the crank and the engine sputtered once, then died.

"This bike is a cold natured bitch," he said as he repeated the procedure. This time the engine started. "I have to warm it up before we take off."

J.P.'s motorcycle engine had a high-pitched sound that reminded Arthur of a sewing machine his mother had when he was a kid. Arthur watched as J.P. climbed on his bike and took off down the dirt road. He revved up the engine and let out on the clutch lever quickly. The front tire of the bike came off the road and he rode for several hundred yards on the rear wheel before he let the front tire come back down to the road.

"J.P. always gets to show off first," Sean said as he took off down the road behind him.

Sean did the same as J.P. had. He rode on the back wheel as far as he could before he brought it back down.

Arthur felt the pride well up in him as he watched Sean ride so well. Most of the worries he had harbored about Sean's riding motorcycles quickly disappeared. Sean was good, but then he had a good teacher. J.P. might do some things that would seem reckless to someone who was not a motorcycle rider, but Arthur knew that he would not be careless. He would be sure his ability would match what he did. He would make sure that Sean knew that, too.

J.P. and Sean turned around and drove back down the road. They reached Arthur at the same time.

"Are we going to ride, or what?"

"Aren't we going to wait for the others to get here?" Arthur asked Sean and J.P.

"Hell no. They will find us. If they don't, we'll come back in a little while to see if they made it," Sean shouted over the noise of the three motorcycles.

"Let's ride!" J.P. yelled as he took off down the dirt road again.

Sean went after him, and Arthur brought up the rear. They rode for a mile down the road before J.P. turned on a trail that was in the curve of the road. Sean and Arthur followed him off the road and onto the trail. The trail was probably made by deer as they headed for water. It was narrow and was surrounded by trees and bushes with long thorns hanging from them. Several of the thorns tore at their clothes as they passed them. They had been on the trail for less than a quarter of a mile before J.P. then stopped. Sean and Arthur pulled up beside him.

"What's the matter?" Sean asked.

"Do you remember him?" J.P. asked.

Sean and Arthur looked and saw the big bull with one crooked horn standing directly in the middle of the trail.

"What do we do now?" Arthur wondered.

"I don't know about you two, but I'm going around him," J.P. said as he took off through the trees around the bull and back on the trail.

The bull ran off the trail toward J.P., and Sean and Arthur took that opportunity to ride down the trail where the bull had been standing. Arthur looked over his shoulder and saw the bull had stopped running. Arthur laughed and waved goodbye to him.

The roots of the tall pine and oak trees grew out onto the trail, and many of them were covered by the pine straw and leaves that had fallen as winter came. Arthur learned his first lesson when he hit one of the large roots. His front tire stopped immediately, his rear tire didn't. The sudden stop sent the back of the motorcycle forward and he went flying over the handlebars and crashing to the ground.

Sean and J.P. immediately turned around and came back. "Are you all right, Mr. Billings?" J.P. shouted as he dropped his bike to the ground and ran to help him.

"Yes, I'm fine," Arthur answered. "I'm just glad I got the first wreck out of the way. Now I won't worry so much about it."

"That's the way to look at it," Sean said.

"Are you sure you are okay, Mr. Billings?" J.P. asked as he helped Arthur pick up his bike.

"I'm great. But please call me Arthur."

They took off down the trail again. This time Arthur watched for everything on the trail ahead of him. He kept Sean's white fender in sight at all times. J.P. was right when he said it would be easy to get lost in these woods. As they reached the top of a long incline in the trail, Arthur noticed that Sean and J.P. had stopped at the top to wait for him. He decided that it was his turn to show off. He revved his engine up and downshifted to second gear and headed straight for them. When he came within fifty feet of them, he slammed on his brakes and leaned to his left. Instead of stopping next to them in an upright position, the bike lay all the way down and slid on its side past them.

"I meant to do that," Arthur said before he even stopped sliding.

"I forgot to tell you something else about those street tires, Mr. Billings," J.P. said.

"What would that be?"

"They don't get any traction on pine straw, either."

"Anything else I should know about these tires, or anything else?" Arthur asked.

"Not that I can think of. If there is, I'm sure you'll find out about them before the day is over."

"I'm sure I will."

After they topped the hill, they came to another trail and took off down it. This one was even narrower than the last one. There were small mounds of dirt that formed a sort of a ramp in the middle of the trail. As he came to the first one, Arthur remembered one of the instructions Sean, or was it J.P., had given him. He was supposed to downshift as he climbed the hill and let the clutch lever out quickly as he went over it. That would make the front tire come up into mid-air and cause the bike to jump over the hill. The first time Arthur tried it, it worked perfectly. The next time was a little more complicated. As he topped the hill, he saw two trees in the trail ahead of him. There was not enough space for the handlebars to pass between them. Arthur turned the handlebars in mid-air at a sharp angle until he passed between the two trees. Then he straightened them out. When he landed on the ground in an upright position, he saw Sean and J.P. sitting on their bikes applauding him.

"That's the way to do it!" J.P. said.

"Yep, we may just make a great dirt bike rider out of you yet!" Sean said with pride showing in his voice.

"I'll settle for just being able to keep up," Arthur laughed.

****

James, Jack and John continued following the trail of blood drops. There were not as many as there had been before, and there was not as much blood as there had been in the beginning. Jack began to suspect that his first instinct was right. They were being led into a trap. They were being baited with less and less bait with each step they took. He suspected it, but he dared not mention it to his father again. He would not be so lucky this time. The way his father was behaving, he might even shoot him if he argued with him again. Jack knew that he could not count on John for support, either. If their father said the sun was blue and there was a bright green stripe running through it, John would swear that he saw that stripe, too. Jack knew he had no choice, all he could do was to go along with this farce. Maybe, if he was lucky, he would spot the man before they reached him. He quit looking for the blood drops on the trail ahead of him. He began looking for the man behind every tree and bush ahead of him.

John saw the blood drop and noticed the way it splattered. He remembered something he had seen on Court TV during the O.J. Simpson trial. There had been an expert witness who testified that blood splatters a different way during different movements as it lands on a surface. If he remembered correctly, the blood drop he was looking at now was caused from blood being dropped from a person going in the left direction, not straight ahead. He cursed himself for not remembering the testimony sooner. Jack was right. The man was leading them where he wanted them to go. But the tables would be turned on the man. Because now John knew what he was doing, and what direction he was heading. He almost called out to his father and Jack to tell them about his discovery, but he changed his mind. He would follow the drops the way he knew the man was going and come up behind him. He would be a hero in his father's eyes when he put a bullet in the man and dragged his body back and dropped it at his father's feet.

John waited until he was sure that his father and Jack were not looking in his direction before he slipped into the trees and followed the trail of blood.

****

Thomas was barely a hundred feet behind the younger boy when he ducked into the woods. The boy had figured out his plan. That was unfortunate, for the boy anyway. Thomas had been following them and waiting for his chance to get to them. The boy made it easy for him. He could take the boy first and come back for the other two.

CHAPTER 8

"Where is John?" Jack asked.

"How the Hell do I know? I'm not his keeper."

"You're his father."

"SO WHAT? I can't keep my eyes on him every minute!" James yelled.

"He was right over there a few minutes ago," Jack anxiously said.

"Maybe the man got him," James offered. "Maybe you were right."

Jack ran past his father and searched the woods and called out for his brother. There was no sign of John, and no answer, either.

"I can't find him. He must have gone off by himself to find the man," Jack said with dread.

"Why would he do a fool thing like that?" James demanded to know.

"To please his father, maybe."

"Could be. Though I didn't think the wimp had it in him," James said.

"He's not a wimp," Jack hissed.

"The hell he's not! I've spent most of my life taking him to the doctor. Him and your mother both."

"You leave my mother out of this! She can't help being sick any more than John can," Jack stated.

"I know. She is constantly telling me that. Why couldn't John and your mother be like you and me? Strong and healthy. I don't think either of us has ever been sick a day in our life," James added.

"We have to go and look for John. If he meets up with that man, there's no telling what will happen," Jack said with urgency.

"John'll probably get his head bashed in," James said.

"And that thought doesn't bother you, Dad?"

"Not particularly. I can't afford the doctor bills anymore. When I lost my job, I also lost my health insurance. And speaking of that, do you want to know the real reason I lost my job?"

"You said they were cutting back," Jack replied.

"Sure. That's what they told me. But I don't believe it. I think the real reason was because your brother and mother's medical bills were making everyone else's insurance premium go up."

"It wouldn't have had anything to do with your drinking, now would it,Dad?" Jack asked with disgust.

"Watch what you say, boy! I just might bash your head in before that lunatic gets a chance to."

"**What kind of a father are you**?" Jack demanded to know.

"The kind I should have been all along," James answered his son.

"**You're more like an animal**."

"That's where you are wrong. If an animal has a weak child, they kill it when it is born because they know it will save the baby from enduring great pain. An animal knows that the weak child will not survive on its own. I should have done that to your brother the day he was born, and to your mother when she first began to get sick all the time," James stated and shrugged.

Jack knew it was useless to argue with his father. He could tell that his speech was becoming more and more slurred with each drink he took. If John was going to be saved, he would have to do it all by himself.

The humming sounds of the motorcycles filled the woods as they looked down the hill and saw the three bikes following the trail beneath them.

"I think I'll do a little target shooting," James said as he raised his rifle and pointed it at the last bike in the row. He lined up the cross-hairs of the scope on the chest of the third rider on the smallest motorcycle. His finger wrapped around the trigger and squeezed just as the rider topped the small mound of dirt.

****

John followed the drops of blood and climbed the hill and faced the bushes. He was going to turn right down the narrow trail when he saw the tiny drop of blood at the base of the bushes. He saw another drop beneath the larger of the bushes. He parted the bushes and saw the doorway to the bunker. It was almost perfectly camouflaged by the thick bushes. If he had not noticed the tiny drop of blood, he would have passed it by completely. His father was going to be extra proud of him for finding this place.

In spite of the cold wind, John had to wipe sweat from his brow. His heart pounded in his chest from the excitement. Or was it fear? It didn't matter at this moment. He took a deep breath and let it out before he slipped between the bushes and stepped inside the bunker. He wrapped his finger around the trigger and gripped the stock of his rifle tightly.

As he stepped inside the bunker, the smell of urine and excrement filled his nostrils. The thrill of the hunt made him ignore the stench. The bunker was dark, but there was enough light coming from the slight openings between the bushes so that he could make out certain things in the bunker. He could see the bones lying in one corner, and he could see the outline of something hanging on the far wall. He waited for his eyes to adjust to the darkness before he took another step. The wounded man could be hiding in one of the dark corners that his vision could not reach.

John felt the warmth from the smoldering fire and tossed a log on it. Within seconds the blaze was roaring and lit up the entire bunker.

John reeled in terror as he saw what was hanging on the far wall. The wall had a line stretched from one end of the bunker to the other. Hanging on that line was meat of all sizes. There were a small deer and two rabbits. The bodies of the animals were not what caused John to gag. Hanging next to the animals were the bodies of two people. A male and a female. The male's body had the arms and legs missing. Their faces were shriveled and an ashen color.

John backed up and tripped over his own feet. His rifle went sliding across the concrete floor of the bunker. He fell backward onto the floor and looked at the rack above the fire. He knew where the male's legs and arms had gone. One of the arms and one of the legs were cooking on the rack above the fire.

He leaned on his side and threw up. His breath came in short rapid gasps. He fumbled in his pocket for his inhaler. He finally got it out and flipped the cap open. He had it inches from his face when it was kicked from his hand. He crawled toward it and was picked up and thrown against the wall. He looked up into the eyes of the man he had been searching for all morning.

"Do you need this?" Thomas asked him as he picked up the inhaler.

John reached for it, but Thomas jerked it away from him.

"You have to ask me nice for it."

John shook his head "no" furiously. His father had always told him that only weak people and cowards begged.

"Are you sure you don't want it? Your breathing don't sound too good," Thomas observed.

John reached for the inhaler again. Thomas continued to hold it just out of his reach.

"You sure are a stubborn fellow," Thomas said as he looked at the inhaler. "If it was me lying on that floor fighting for every breath, I sure would ask for it."

John tried to calm himself down. So many times, if he concentrated hard enough, the attack would subside. But he had never had one this bad before. He tried anyway. He closed his eyes and tried to put his mind away from this terrible place. He tried to envision a nice red brick home, much like his own, except the parents in that home didn't argue all the time like his parents did. The father in that home didn't drink and complain to his youngest son about how much money his medicine cost. John had no trouble placing his mother's face on the woman in that home, but no matter how hard he tried, he could not put his own father's face on the man in that happy home. His breathing slowed somewhat as the picture came into his mind. He managed that by placing his brother Jack's face on the father in that home. His brother was more of a father to him anyway. He always took care of him and comforted him when he was depressed. Yes, his brother would be a perfect father someday.

The attack was well on its way to subsiding when Thomas's voice shattered his solitude.

"Don't die on me! Not yet, anyway!" Thomas yelled. He had mistaken the slowed breathing of the attack's passing for John dying.

The asthma attack returned immediately to John with more intensity than it had before. He fought for every single breath now. He could not summon the vision that would save his life. He knew deep down in his soul that he was going to die. John made up his mind that he would go out of this world much differently than the way he had come into it. He was born sickly and crying. He would leave this life behind with a bravery that would even make his father proud. He stiffened his back and opened his eyes wide and stared into the face of the man he had hunted. He stopped fighting for each breath.

Thomas looked down on John and saw the arrogance in his eyes. "You are a brave boy. There are not many people that could die so calmly. Unfortunately, you are not one of those people. You will die with fear consuming you until the last beat of your heart."

John shook his head "no" again.

"We shall see, boy. We shall see," Thomas said as he grabbed John's right arm and dragged him across the room to the door of the cage.

John looked through the wire of the cage and instantly lost every bit of the nerve he had acquired. He looked into the savage eyes of the occupant of the cage and he tried to scream a scream that would not come. He tried to move but he was frozen in place. He wasn't sure if it was a result of his attack or if it was because of the terror that racked every fiber of his body. For the first time in his life, John wanted to die. He wanted to die before he was put into the cage. He prayed for death to come to him quickly. This prayer, just like all the others in his life, for him and his mother to get well, was unanswered as Thomas opened the door to the cage and threw him into it.

He felt the teeth tearing into his body before the cage door was closed behind him. He felt the searing pain as big chunks of his flesh were bitten off his arm. He also felt the relief in his spirit as his heart was torn from his chest. Then he felt nothing.

****

"What happened, Dad?" Sean yelled as he stopped his motorcycle and ran back to Arthur.

"I hit another damn root."

"Are you all right?" Sean asked.

"Yes. I guess it just knocked me out for a few seconds when I hit the ground."

"That's not all that happened," J.P. said.

"What!?"

J.P. pointed to the tree where the bullet had hit. The bark was sheared away. He took out his pocket knife and dug the lead slug from the tree.

"I would say a hunter thought you looked like a deer," he said as he tossed the slug to Arthur.

Arthur eyed the slug closely as he rolled it over and over in his hand. It was still warm. He scanned the horizon for a sign of the person who had fired the bullet. He didn't see anything.

"Why don't we ride somewhere else for a while? The hunters will be leaving the woods pretty soon."

"Sounds like a good idea to me. Let's ride back to the camp and see if the others have gotten there yet," Arthur answered.

They got on their bikes and rode back toward the camp. Arthur tried not to let them see the concern on his face. He didn't believe that any hunter, even a blind one could mistake a man on a motorcycle for a deer. He did not enjoy the ride back to camp as much as he did the ride from camp. He was too busy watching every movement in the trees ahead of him, and behind him. He had an uneasy feeling that he could not shake.

****

James was ready to fire another shot at the motorcycle rider when Jack grabbed his arm and took the rifle away from him.

"What are you doing? You could have killed him!" Jack yelled.

"I would have too if he hadn't fallen off his bike," James replied.

"Why?" Jack asked. "We don't even know him. He never did anything to us."

"That doesn't matter to me anymore. I don't like motorcycle riders. I never have, and I never will."

"Are you going to kill everyone you don't like?" Jack demanded to know.

"**I just might**," James responded. "I should warn you that every time you sass me, I like you a little less."

"Do you want to kill me?" Jack demanded to know.

"No, not right now anyway," his father answered.

"What's that supposed to mean?" Jack quickly questioned.

"Oh, you'll see."

"We had better go look for John," Jack said.

He wanted to change the subject. He didn't like the direction this conversation was heading. He handed the rifle back to his father.

"Forget about John. He's probably dead," James instructed.

"Why do you say that?"

"Because if he caught up with that man, he couldn't handle him and he got killed. If he didn't catch up with him, he's so weak that the cold or one of his asthma attacks probably killed him. The way I see it, any way you look at it, John is dead."

"I don't believe that! And, dear Dad, if it were true, you don't look too upset about it!"

"I'm not," James said in a cold way.

"How can you say that about your own son?"

"You would be surprised at what I can say, or do. I was hoping that John or you, or both of you for that matter, would have been killed last night by that man in the camp," James informed him.

"He wasn't after us! He was after you," Jack said with hatred.

"That's true, but I didn't know that until he attacked my tent," his father answered.

"You knew he was out there?"

"Of course, I did. Why do you think I wasn't in my tent? I slipped out under the side and hid behind the car until he came running into the camp," James continued.

Jack thought for a moment. "Are you saying that if he had attacked our tent you would not have stopped him?"

"That's exactly what I'm saying. I would have killed him after he killed you two. But he surprised me and went after my tent, and I didn't aim good enough, I guess," James said with certainty.

Jack took a step backward. He was trying to convince himself that his father didn't mean a word of what he was saying, that it was the booze talking. Deep in his heart he knew that wasn't it. He had seen his father drunk many times over his lifetime. Never had the alcohol made him so cruel and vicious.

"Why would you want him to kill us?" Jack asked the question, but he wasn't sure he wanted to know the answer.

"To save me the trouble. I wasn't sure I could do it," his father informed him.

"Why do you want us dead?"

"Because it's over, all over," James responded with no feeling.

"What's over? Talk to me Dad."

"Our life, that's what. Our family. It's all finished," James explained.

"You are ready to give up on living just because you lost your job? You said yourself that other companies would be begging you to come to work for them."

"I lied," James said. "No one wants me anymore."

"You are wrong about that, Dad. I want you, John loves you more than anything, and Mom couldn't live without you."

"How did you know about that?" James demanded.

"About what, Dad? How did I know about what?"

"About your mother."

"What about her?"

"She's dead," James announced.

"You're lying!" Jack yelled.

"I'm afraid not. I killed her yesterday morning right before

84

we left the house to come up here. I smothered her with a pillow."

Jack dropped to his knees on the ground and the tears flowed from his eyes. He believed his father. Even in his worst drunken stupor, he could not concoct a story like this. He looked at his father, the man he had admired all his life. Jack realized at this very moment that he never really knew his father.

"Why? Why did you do it?"

"For a lot of reasons. I guess the main one was because she was sick all of the time. I just got tired of it," James said with no regret.

"Are you sure it wasn't for more selfish reasons?"

"What do you mean by that?"

"Maybe you were the weak one, not her. Maybe you were not strong enough to handle her illness. She handled it pretty good for a woman who was in constant pain," Jack said with sadness.

"I'm not weak. Your brother and her were the weak ones," his father sneered.

"I don't think so. I think you are weak. Too weak to handle the disappointments in life. Too weak to accept that you lost your job to a younger, and maybe more qualified person."

"You had better be careful of what you're saying."

"Not anymore, Dad. I've been watching what I've been saying around you all my life. Well, I'm tired of being careful of what I say! And I'm tired of doing everything to please you."

"**I'm warning you**!" James yelled.

"What are you going to do, Dad? Kill me like you did Mom? That's why you brought us out here, isn't it? To kill us. Or were you going to just kill John because you thought he was like Mom? You thought he was weak, too. Well I've got news for you! Mom was not weak and neither was John! They both faced their illnesses with more bravery than you will ever have. Do you think you could go through what they went through and still manage to find a bright side to everything? I can answer that question for you. You couldn't even begin to handle it. You couldn't face every day like they did. You couldn't handle the rejection you showed them. John was so hungry for you to accept him that he was willing to kill for that acceptance. If he is dead, I hope he died before he became what you wanted him to become."

"You know what? In the beginning, when we first arrived here, I was a little sad because I had to kill you. I'm not sad about that anymore. You just showed me that you are not strong either. I wish you could see yourself like I'm seeing you. A grown man crying in the dirt. You are no son of mine," James said with disgust.

"I wish to God I wasn't! I wish I would have died before I found out what kind of man you really are."

"You'll get part of that wish soon. Very soon. After we hunt that man down and kill him."

"You must be crazy if you think I'm going anywhere with you!"

"I am crazy. That's what the company doctors said. They said that I had some kind of chemical imbalance. They suspect it was caused by years of alcohol abuse. They wanted me to take medical leave."

"Then they didn't fire you, they just wanted to help you," Jack said with dismay.

"How? By putting me in a mental hospital?"

"If that's what it took to make you well," Jack answered.

"I am well, damn it! They are the ones that are sick. Every damn one of them. I told the two company doctors that. I even told the president of the company that. Right before I killed them."

"You killed them, too?" Jack asked in disbelief.

"I sure did. I showed them who was sick. If I was sick, that meant I was weak. I'm not weak. They were weak. They begged on their hands and knees for their lives. But I was strong. I didn't let their pitiful cries for mercy sway me in my decision. I was strong and carried out my duty like a man."

"**You are not a man**. I don't know what you are, but you are not human."

"You are entitled to your opinion, although, if I were you I would not voice it too often around me."

"The police will be looking for you. They will come up here to find you."

"No, they won't," James answered. "At least not until Monday. That's when the secretary will discover the bodies in the office. Then they will go to our house and find your mother. I left a note telling them where to find us. Of course, by the time they get here, you and I will be dead, too. They will find the body of the man from last night next to us. That will be a little added bonus for them. I'm sure he's wanted for something."

"**You are insane!!**" Jack yelled.

"Yes, I guess I am. Now get up and let's hunt that son-of-a-bitch down and kill him so we can die in peace."

"I won't go!"

"Yes, you will. You know what? I'm really disappointed in you, son. I didn't expect you to take it nearly this hard. I expected you to be a little upset, but not hysterical. You remind me of your little brother."

"I consider that a compliment."

"Still trying to push me over the edge, aren't you?" James asked.

"I would love to push you over the edge of a cliff!"

"That's the Jack I know. Now get up and let's go. I won't tell you again."

"No!"

"That did it. I'm tired of fucking around with you."

James raised his rifle and fired without even taking aim. The bullet hit Jack directly between his eyes. A small trickle of blood ran down his forehead as he fell face first onto the ground.

He walked over and stood over Jack's body. He felt no remorse or sadness as he looked down on the body of his son. Jack was in a much better place than this stinking world. He was with his mother in a place where she felt no pain. More than likely, his brother John was there, too. He could hardly wait to find the man and kill him. The sooner that task was done, the sooner James knew he could join his family. They would all be together again in a place where there were no doctor bills, no trips to the emergency room at the hospital, and best of all, no reason to be brave.

****

Thomas stood and watched the events as they unfolded before him. He could hear every word and see every action. He saw and heard it all, but he wasn't sure he could believe it. How could a man kill his own son in cold blood like James just did? He had seen James try to shoot the motorcycle rider. That he could easily understand. All the motorcycle riders did was to make noise and disturb the peace and quiet of the forest. But to kill his own son. James Foster was a truly evil man. A man who possessed such evil did not belong in his woods. He had to rid the woods of such an evil influence. Thomas had planned on killing the man from the beginning for invading his woods. Now, he had another reason to do it. He would kill James Foster for not only trespassing, but he would also kill him for revenge. Thomas would take the revenge that Jack could not.

Thomas would not be careless again as he had been last night. He would be even more careful when he hunted James Foster now that he knew he was dealing with a madman. Such a man would be unpredictable. He would not do what was expected. He would be irrational in his actions. Thomas knew that James Foster would be his most challenging quarry. It would be the most exciting, yet the most enjoyable, when the moment came and he killed James. The excitement of the hunt to come welled up in Thomas and spread through his entire body. Something else came over Thomas, too. Another emotion mingled in with the thrill of the hunt. That emotion was apprehension. For the first time in his entire life, Thomas feared someone.

CHAPTER 9

Sean, J.P., and Arthur rounded the last curve in the road before they reached their campsite. They saw a car and two pickup trucks parked at the edge of the road. The crowd of people who were unloading their motorcycles greeted them as they pulled up beside them. Arthur counted eight people as he followed J.P. and Sean and parked his motorcycle next to the Suburban.

Sean had barely gotten off his motorcycle when a huge, fat girl ran over to him and threw her arms around him and kissed him deeply on the lips. Sean pushed her gently away.

"I didn't know you were coming," Sean said as he stole a quick glance in Arthur's direction.

"I haven't seen you in over a month. What was I supposed to do, sit around the house forever and wait until you decided to call or come over?" she demanded to know.

Arthur did his best to conceal the surprise and slight anger from his face. He got off his bike and began checking the tightness of his chain. It was an action he did for no other reason than to hide his face in case his efforts to disguise his disgust at the sight of the girl failed.

The girl's name was Angela. She made everyone call her Angel. Each time Arthur heard someone call her that, he had to stifle a loud scream. He couldn't help but think how outrageous it was to call what he considered the epitome of evil, an Angel. She and Sean had been dating on and off for about two years, and Arthur despised her. At one point Sean and Angela were engaged. This dating relationship had caused the only major friction between Arthur and Sean. Angela was the only chink in the armor of the relationship between Arthur and his son. Arthur had not liked her from the first day he had met her. He tried to tell himself that it was not just because she was fat and the flab hung from her arms and quivered when she walked. Whenever the weather was warm enough she always wore sleeveless T-shirts. Arthur was glad it was cold outside today. She had to wear a large windbreaker. He knew that was a major part of his dislike for her. How could she expect anyone else to respect her when she didn't respect herself enough to take care of her body. Arthur also disliked her because she drank too much. And when Sean was around her he drank too much, too. Arthur suspected that the glazed look she always had in her eyes was a sign of drug use, too. As far as Arthur knew, that particular habit of hers had not infected Sean. Arthur was convinced in his mind that Angela was just after Sean to trap him into marrying her.

Angela had ridden up to the woods in Terry Richardson's truck. Terry was a casual friend of Sean's. Arthur liked most of Sean's friends. But he didn't like Terry. There was no doubt that Terry was a drunk and a drug user. He had been arrested twice for driving while under the influence of alcohol and had also been busted several times for possession of drugs. If his uncle were not a judge, he would be in prison instead of on probation. Terry was built like a body builder. His shoulders were broad, and muscles rippled underneath the flannel shirt he wore. Arthur figured that Terry must possess a body that thrived naturally in spite of the abuse that his alcohol and drug use cast upon it.

Arthur watched Angela and Sean out of the corner of his eye as they walked past him. She was dressed in tight blue jeans that did nothing for her except reveal the fact her butt was so fat that it had no curve to it. The tight jeans also made her body appear to have a bell shape to it. As usual, Angela's make-up was complete and her long, dark colored hair was styled to perfection. Arthur disliked the girl so much that he held that against her, too. It was ridiculous for her to be made up as if she were going out to the theater when she was going motorcycle riding in the woods. Before the day was over, her face would be covered with mud, and the new designer jeans that she wore would be torn from the briars and limbs that lined the trails. To be fair to her, Arthur did admit that she had a pretty face. That was the only positive thing he could say about her. As far as Arthur was concerned, her many negatives overshadowed that one positive trait.

Arthur couldn't understand what Sean saw in Angela. Arthur refused to call her Angel. Sean was an extremely good looking young man and could have any girl he wanted, but he always seemed to be attracted to fat ones. Arthur had tried to analyze it once. He had come to three conclusions. First, Sean had a low self-esteem problem and didn't believe that he was handsome enough for the good looking women. That was a little hard for Arthur to accept because Sean had dated many good-looking women in his short lifetime. The second reason he had come up with was that extremely obese women, like Angela, were so starved for attention from such a good-looking guy like Sean that they would do anything he wanted them to do sexually. The final reason Arthur had come up with was that Sean liked fat women because he did not have to worry about them fooling around on him. And if they caught him fooling around on them, they were quick to forgive and forget. This was the reason that Arthur tended to believe more than the other two because Angela had caught Sean on several occasions going out with other girls, even as recently as last month with the last one, and here she was hanging on to him like a tick would hang onto a fat dog. " Did you miss your little Angel?" she asked Sean as she wrapped her arms around him.

Arthur fooled with his chain with even more ferocity.

"We'll talk about everything later," Sean answered as he glanced over at his father.

Sean knew how Arthur felt about Angela, and he was angry with her for coming to the woods. He didn't want anything to spoil the weekend with his father.

Arthur turned his head away from Angela and Sean as he pulled on his chain and let it spring back.

"Excuse me, Mr. Billings, but we don't have an extra chain. If you keep that up, you might just break that chain with your bare hands," J.P. said over Arthur's shoulder.

Arthur looked up at him and smiled. His anger had begun to fade as quickly as it had come.

"I'm just checking it. I got a limb tangled up in it earlier."

"I don't know about that. For a minute, I thought you were going to bite it in two. Your face looked to be twice as tight as that chain."

Arthur laughed and his anger faded completely. J.P. had showed him in his own special way that he should put away his animosity and anger for today.

"I guess it's fine," Arthur said as he stood up. "In fact, everything is fine now. And call me Arthur."

"I'm glad to hear that," J.P. said smiling.

"J.P., come over here and look at this for me," the voice belonged to Terry Richardson.

J.P. began to walk away. Arthur called him back.

"Thanks, J.P.. I appreciate your help," Arthur said as he extended his hand and J.P. shook it firmly.

"No problem. The chain is fine," J.P. said as he walked away.

Arthur didn't get a response from J.P. and he didn't expect one. J.P. was that kind of a person. He minded his own business, but if he could help defuse the tension around him, he didn't hesitate to help.

Arthur lit a cigarette and watched as J.P. got a screwdriver and began to adjust the carburetor on Terry's bike. It was an on/off road bike. It had the suspension for trail riding, but it had all the safety features, such as headlights and turn signals, for street riding. As Arthur watched he remembered that Sean told him Terry was a lousy dirt rider. Arthur had no doubt that the taillights and headlights, as well as a few other things, would be torn from the bike by the end of the day. Within a minute after he began twisting the small screw, J.P. had the engine that had been sputtering and groaning purring like a newborn kitten.

Arthur watched as J.P. went to the next motorcycle, a red three wheeler that belonged to Joe and Nancy Petrie. Arthur knew them well. They were two people who had grown up in the same neighborhood Arthur lived in, and they were always together. When they eloped a few weeks ago, it came as no surprise to Arthur. They fell in love the first day they met in preschool, and that love had not faltered for a moment since then.

As J.P. reached around for a wrench, Sean handed it to him as if he had read his mind.

"Twelve millimeter."

"You have come a long way," J.P. said.

"I've got a good teacher," Sean answered.

J.P. had only a few adjustments to make on the three-wheeler before he was through.

"Anybody else?" J.P. asked.

"My Honda 225 is running perfectly," Mark Helms said. "Since I rebuilt the motor I haven't had a bit of trouble out of it."

Arthur didn't doubt that, either. Mark was an extremely good mechanic. Between Mark and J.P., Arthur never had to worry about his riding lawn mower, his weed-eater, or his cars being broken down for long. Neither Mark nor J.P. would ever willingly accept money for repairing something. Arthur had to force them to take any money for their work. Sometimes they would even argue playfully over who was going to fix something if it broke. They would argue over fixing everything except Arthur's Mustang. J.P. was a Chevrolet man and hated to work on Fords. He always said that "Ford" meant "Found on Russian Dump." He would gripe and complain when the Mustang needed repairs, but he would always fix it. Mark, on the other hand, loved Ford vehicles, and Arthur had sat and listened to them for many nights as they sat around the supper table and traded insults about the differences between Chevrolet and Ford.

Arthur considered himself extremely lucky to have these two young men in his life. Not because he would never have to pay for another repair, but because they were like extra sons. They always showed him and his wife Elizabeth the utmost respect. J.P. had needed a little training in the beginning when he would let the "F" word slip out every now and then in front of Elizabeth, but he was doing much better at watching what he said.

Mark had brought Tiffanie Simon with him. She was a short, lovely girl with long dark hair. She did not wear any make-up, and she wore heavy jeans and a big sweatshirt that hid her firm figure and ample breasts. Arthur liked her a lot. She always had a friendly smile for everyone.

"My brakes are not working right," Damuth said.

Damuth Hendricks was another friend who had grown up in the neighborhood with Sean. He was always a good kid and managed to never get involved in the minor trouble that Sean and a few of the other kids in the neighborhood had when they were growing up. Damuth had brought Gerard Bradley with him. Arthur had met Gerard a few times when he came to the house with Damuth. Arthur wondered if there was a closer relationship between these two young men than a mere friendship. Damuth was not very masculine. His features were soft and Arthur had never seen him play any rough sports. Riding motorcycles was the roughest thing he had ever seen him do. As far as Arthur knew, Damuth had never had a date with a girl, and he never heard either of them talk about girls. It didn't set well with Arthur that they might be gay, but he would never say anything that would hurt either of them. They could live their lives the way they wanted to, just as Arthur lived his life the way he wanted to. He had no right to try to challenge their decision any more than they had a right to change his.

As Arthur watched Sean hand J.P. the tools to adjust the brakes on the motorcycle, he could tell from the pleasure on J.P.'s face that he did not feel like he was being taken advantage of. J.P. realized that he had been born with a natural aptitude to work on engines, and he had developed that talent by studying and learning everything he could to enhance that talent. He felt a sense of duty to do everything he could to make everyone's motorcycle as safe as possible while they were engaged in one of the most dangerous recreational sports there was.

Arthur considered telling J.P. or Sean that his brakes were not working as well as they had when he first began to ride this morning. On the way back to the campsite he had to push twice as hard to get them to grab. He decided against saying anything even though they had told him that they may have to make some minor adjustments along the trail because his motorcycle had not been driven hard in such a long time. They had told him that some things would loosen and others would tighten as he rode and not to hesitate to say something. J.P. and Sean had worked long and hard on his motorcycle to get it ready for Christmas Eve. He would not put any more burdens on them to work on it now. As long as the brakes were grabbing, and they didn't get any worse, he would remain silent about them.

CHAPTER 10

James Foster left his son lying in the dirt and went through the woods. He threw away the extra bottle of bourbon in his knapsack. He did not need anything that would dull his senses as he tracked the man from the night before. He surprised himself at the ease of throwing the bourbon away. It had not bothered him at all. He began to wonder if he could have, or should have, done it years ago. He couldn't help but wonder if things would be different if he had. He didn't dwell on that scenario for very long. It didn't matter. The past was gone, and no matter what he did now or how much he hoped that things would be different, they could not be changed. The present was here, and he had to accept it. None of that mattered at this very moment. The one thing that did matter was that he had to find the man and kill him. It would be the last act he would do before he died, either by his own hand or as a result of any wounds he would sustain in the battle with the man that had attacked the camp last night.

James continued through the woods and listened carefully. He was disappointed when he did not hear the sounds of the motorcycles. It would please him if he could take one or two of them out with his rifle before he found the old man. It would be good practice. He still cursed himself for missing the rider earlier. He wondered if the rider had a guardian angel riding on his shoulder with him. James discounted that thought quickly. From the quick glimpse he had gotten of the rider when he removed his helmet, James could tell that he was older than the other two he was with. Much older. The rider was probably trying to recapture his youth and that made James hate him even more. Once gone, youth is one thing that cannot be recovered. Any man that thought it could be was a fool, and fools did not deserve to live. A split second was all that separated the rider from life and death. Earlier today, time had been on the rider's side. If James saw him again, that would change. Time would be on his side.

****

Thomas followed closely behind James, but not too closely. The sound of a snapping twig underneath his feet might be heard by James, and he would know he was being followed. That was one thing that Thomas did not want James to know. From the bits of conversation Thomas had heard, James thought that he was running for his life. Thomas did not want to do anything that would alter that idea in James' mind. Thomas was already disappointed when he saw him throw the bottle away. He had secretly hoped that he would drink all of it, get drunk and pass out, or at least stop to sleep it off. That would have made everything so easy. Things did not come easy for Thomas, so he did not dwell on his disappointment. He would wait. He would be patient. He did not know when, or how, he would kill James, but he would wait until the opportunity presented itself. Then he would seize upon it and exact the vengeance that was rightfully his. Thomas would share that vengeance with the spirit of the man's son.

****

A slow, drizzling rain began falling as J.P. and Sean finished fixing the brakes on Damuth's motorcycle. The biting cold was intensified as the water collected and soaked through their clothes.

"Is everybody ready?" Sean asked to all of them, but no one in particular. "Watch out for the deer hunters. One of them almost killed my old man earlier."

Everyone answered with the same gesture. They started the engines on their motorcycles and revved them up at the same time. The result was a deafening sound that filled the woods around them.

Arthur started his engine and drove slowly over next to Sean and stopped when he saw Angela get on the back of Terry's bike.

"I don't care if she rides with you," Arthur said as he motioned toward Angela.

"I told her I didn't invite her up here to ride. She came with Terry, so she can ride with him."

"I really don't mind. It's okay," Arthur repeated as he tried to convince Sean he was sincere even though he knew in his heart that he wasn't.

"Listen to me, Dad. Watch my lips. This trip was for you and me. Not her. I'm sick of her trying to interfere and come between us. She wouldn't like the trails we are going to ride on anyway. All she would do is bitch and gripe about the mud and briars."

"Are you sure?" Arthur asked.

"Yes, I'm positive. Now let's ride," Sean said without hesitation.

The sound of J.P.'s engine would have drowned out any answer or further argument Arthur could have given. He was glad that it did. He saw Angela's make-up as the rain hit her face and her mascara began to run in long black streaks down her chubby cheeks and onto her neck. He stifled a smile. He also saw the hurt expression on Sean's face as Angela wrapped her arms tightly around Terry's waist as they took off. A twinge of guilt passed through him and erased his smile. Sean was a good son. Arthur wanted to be a good father to Sean. He made up his mind that when this trip was over, he would try to accept Angela, or at least keep his opinion of her to himself. Sean was a grown man and had to live his own life. Arthur finally realized that fact. It was odd that the reality had come to him as he sat on a motorcycle in a freezing rain in the middle of the woods. He wondered if there was something special about these woods. He wondered if there was a presence that existed in these woods that gnawed at a man's soul and made him look within himself and see what no other person, including himself, could see. Arthur smelled the air. The rain seemed to wash away the smell of the gasoline and the exhausts immediately and cleanse the air. It was a fresh smell, a smell that brought peace and tranquility to him. Arthur also sensed something else in the air and the woods that surrounded him. He didn't know what it was, but it gave him a sense of foreboding and sent chills up and down his spine even more than the rain and the cold did. He forced that feeling away. He was with his son and J.P. What could go wrong?

As Arthur watched the others ride away through the woods in all different directions, he tried to feel truly happy.

"We aren't all going to ride together?" he asked J.P.

"No, we are not."

"Why not?" Arthur asked. "None of them know their way around these woods, either."

"They all want to do their own thing," J.P. answered. "Joe and Nancy's three-wheeler can't fit between the trees on most of the trails we ride on, and Joe and Nancy are probably going to find a nice cozy place and make love. They like to do it in the outdoors. They are kind of kinky that way."

"What about Damuth and Gerard?" Arthur wondered out loud.

"They are more than likely going to do the same thing, with a little variation, of course," J.P. answered.

"I would prefer not to hear about that," Arthur stated.

"I don't even want to think about it," J.P. said.

"What about Angela and Terry? I figured she would want to be right on Sean's ass," Arthur commented.

"She probably would love that. But Terry can't handle the trails and hills we are going to ride on and he knows it. He doesn't want to be made to look like the lousy rider he is in front of her. They will probably find a trail for themselves. He's been trying to get into her drawers for a long time."

"The only way I would want to get into her drawers is if I shit in mine," Arthur said.

"They wouldn't fit!" J.P. laughed.

"What about Mark? He's a good rider. He could take the trails we did."

"Yes, he could, with no problem," J.P. agreed. "But he's got Tiffanie with him. He'll try to find a cozy place, too."

"Why the hell did they come out here in the freezing cold?" Arthur asked. "They would have all been better off going to a motel. At least they would have been warm."

"I don't think any of them will have any trouble getting warm. At least not for a while," J.P. said as he revved up his engine and took off on the rear wheel.

Sean took off right behind him, and Arthur followed them. As he rode into the woods and followed them down a trail that seemed narrower than the one they had taken earlier, Arthur remembered a few times when he was younger that he had taken girls riding in the woods. He didn't blame any of them for going their own way. He was young once himself. At this very moment he didn't feel old at all. He felt younger than any of them and secretly wished that Elizabeth had come with him. He wouldn't mind finding them a trail they could make love on, too.

****

Thomas stopped and rested each time James did. He was beginning to enjoy this little game. It lent excitement to a life that he had missed since the military base closed. He used to follow the soldiers, too. That was even more challenging because when he killed them, he always had to make it look like an accident. That had taken careful planning on his part. Thomas remembered all the unique plans he had devised. A rattlesnake in a sleeping bag had worked perfectly for a few of the soldiers. A dead tree pushed down at the precise moment had been good for at least two more of them. Once he had even bashed a soldier's head in with a rock and rolled him off one of the cliffs that were at the top of a steep hill. None of the deaths were ever suspected of being anything but what they all appeared to be, accidents.

When he first overheard the conversations of the soldiers and learned the base was being closed because of budget cutbacks, he had to stifle a laugh or they would have heard him. He had been sitting in a tree right above their heads. He almost laughed out loud because he knew that he had won the war he had declared on the United States Military. He didn't believe the reasons they talked about for the closing of the base. He knew in his heart that it was because they were afraid. They were afraid of an unseen, and unknown, enemy that was slowly depleting their ranks. They would leave his woods because he had beaten them in the battle for his woods.

A sound behind him made Thomas jump. He turned quickly and stood face to face with James Foster. He had become so engrossed in his thoughts that he had been careless and had taken his eyes off of him.

"I knew I would get you sooner or later, but I didn't think it would be this easy," James said as he raised his rifle and pointed it toward Thomas's chest.

"You have not gotten me yet," Thomas said calmly.

"What do you call this?" James asked with irritation.

"All I see is a cold-blooded killer with a rifle," Thomas calmly replied.

"You are calling me a killer? What do you think you are? You tried to cave in my skull last night," James responded.

"I had a reason to kill you. You kill for no reason at all. You even killed your own son," Thomas accused.

"I kind of had a feeling that you knew about that. I had my reasons. They may not seem important to you, but they are to me."

"There is never a reason for a man to kill his own son," Thomas exclaimed.

"That doesn't matter now!" James shouted angrily. "What does matter is that you are going to die. Right now."

Thomas watched calmly as James aimed the rifle at his chest. He did not show any fear or any other emotion as he watched James's finger tighten around the trigger. He would either live or die. Whatever was to be, would be.

Thomas waited for the pain that would invade his heart and bring his life's blood forth, gushing to the ground. He was ready to return to the earth.

"Before I shoot you, I want to know one thing," James said. "Why did you try to kill me last night?"

"I had my reasons. They would not seem very important to a man like you," Thomas replied.

"I can live with that. Too bad you can't," James said as he pulled the trigger.

Thomas did not feel the bullet crashing into his chest. He

didn't feel anything. But he did hear something, and it was not the sound of a gunshot. He heard the faint click of the trigger as the gun misfired. He saw the surprised look on James's face and did not give him time to recover. He swung his stick around and knocked the rifle from his hands. He brought the stick around again and it caught James on the side of his head and sent him into a spinning motion to the ground.

He was standing over James with the pointed end of the stick pressed to his throat before he could regain his senses. James had a dazed look on his face.

"I guess I will not die today after all," he told James.

"Go ahead. Do it. I'm not afraid to die. I've planned on it and even looked forward to it," James told him adamantly.

"I know," Thomas said softly. "I know a lot of things about you. I know you planned on killing yourself after you killed me. I know you hate suffering."

"Just do it. Don't bore me to death," James said.

"I'm going to do it," Thomas explained. "But not the way you want it to be."

"Would you please kill me and get it over with?" James pleaded.

"You would like that, wouldn't you? You would like to die quickly and not feel any more pain again."

"Please kill me! I'm begging you!" James cried.

"I will. I promise I will kill you. But not the way you want it. I will kill you in a way that you will have time to think about your life and all the wrongs you have done," Thomas told James softly.

James felt a dread come over him. He had not counted on this. He had assumed that the man was crazy and would kill him the first chance he got. He didn't like the things this man was saying. He didn't have to think about it for long. A swift movement of the man's stick on the side of his head made the sky turn black.

****

"Slow down! You are throwing mud on my new jeans!" Angela yelled.

"Quit your bitching!" Terry yelled back at her. "What did you think we were going to do out here, have a picnic on a nice, clean table?"

"I want to go find Sean. I'll ride with him," Angela whined.

"That's the only reason you came up here, isn't it? To be with Sean. All that talk last night about us was just a lot of conning bullshit," he said in anger.

"I knew you were stupid, but I didn't know you were stupid enough to believe all that stuff I said last night," Angela argued.

Terry slammed on his brakes to avoid a large rut in the trail and lost control of his motorcycle. He and Angela slid off the trail and ended up in the middle of a patch of thorns.

"Damn you! You can't drive worth a shit! You have completely ruined my pants!" Angela shouted as she scrambled back onto the trail and began pulling the thorns out of her arms.

"Help me get my bike out of these things," Terry ordered.

"You put it in there. You get it out."

"If you want some of this stuff I brought with me, you'll help me get it out," Terry said quickly.

Angela ignored the pain from the thorns and didn't let the mud bother her as she helped Terry drag the motorcycle back onto the trail.

He got on it, and after several tries at cranking, had it running again.

"Well, where is it?" she asked.

"Where's what?" Terry asked.

"You know what I'm talking about," Angela said with clinched teeth.

"Oh. The little pleasures I promised I would bring?" Terry questioned Angela.

"Yes. Now stop fooling around with that motorcycle and give me something. My arms hurt from those thorns sticking me," she moaned.

"Dr. Terry has just the thing for what ails you," he said as he killed the engine. He pulled a plastic bag full of colored pills from his jacket pocket and held it in front of her.

Angela's eyes lit up like a Christmas tree in a dark room as she took the bag from his hand and swallowed three of the small red pills.

"Slow down. This stuff ain't cheap. You just took about twenty bucks worth," Terry barked.

"I'm good for it," Angela said.

"We'll see about that before this day is over," Terry said with a slight twinkle in his eye.

****

Thomas picked up James , threw him over his shoulder as if he were a rag doll, and started off toward his bunker. The weight of the man did not bother him too much. Over the years he had carried many things that weighed more. As he went through the bushes that hid his bunker, he heard the noise and stopped. The sounds of the motorcycle engines surrounded him and made it seem as if they were right beside him. Thomas knew they weren't. The sounds were echoing through the still woods and carried far from where they emanated. He did know that there were more than the three he had seen this morning. Three motorcycles were more than he could tolerate. The sounds of many more were more than he could stand. He would take care of James and then put a stop to that infernal noise that shattered the tranquility of his woods.

Thomas carried James into the bunker and laid him down next to the large cage. He took some vines that he had gathered from the woods in case he ever needed string and tied James's hands and feet securely with it. He dipped some water from the stream in a small turtle shell and splashed it onto James's face. James awoke instantly.

"Where am I? Am I dead?"

"You are not that lucky," Thomas said.

"What are you going to do to me? Why have you brought me here?" James asked with fear.

"I wanted you to have the chance to say one last good-bye to your youngest son before you died."

"Where is he?" James asked. Maybe John could help him get away. Suddenly James did not want to die anymore.

"He's right beside you."

James moved his head to the side and saw the half-eaten corpse lying inside the cage. The insides had been torn out and spilled onto the floor. Huge chunks of flesh had been bitten off of many areas of the corpse's arms and legs. If it were not for the look of terror on the unblemished face of his son, James would not have recognized the body as John's. He fought the bile rising from his stomach and swallowed it. Fear began to consume him.

"Please let me go. I swear I won't tell anyone about you, or what you've done," James begged.

"I know you won't. You will never tell anyone anything ever again," Thomas replied.

The sound of the occupant of the cage crashing into the wire to get at James made him scream. James tried to roll away from the cage, but he could move only a few inches. The vines that bound his hands were looped through the wire of the cage.

"You can't just leave me here with that thing. I'll starve to death," James begged again.

"You won't starve. I'll be back long before that happens. And when I return, I'll put you in that cage, just like I did your son. But until that moment, you will have plenty of time to think about what you have done in your lifetime. You will have plenty of time to try and ask God for forgiveness for your sins. I doubt that he will listen to scum like you, but before you die, you will be begging him for mercy."

Thomas left with the sound of James' voice begging him to let him go as he went searching for the motorcycle riders. The task of carrying James to the bunker had tired him, and he was feeling the strain of his years catching up with him. He would dispose of the rest of the trespassers quickly. He would not toy with them. He would have all the entertainment he could stand for one day with James when he returned to the bunker.

Thomas was listening for the sounds of motorcycle engines and heard voices instead. He could tell the people were arguing.

"Why does everyone have to bring their problems and fights

to my woods?" he asked himself as he slipped quietly through the trees toward the sound of the people arguing.

"I want to go find Sean!" Angela screamed in a high-pitched voice.

"I'm not going out in those woods. I've found a nice safe trail, and I'm going to ride on it," Terry responded.

"If you want it so safe, why did you come up here?" she asked.

"It was your idea to come up here, remember?" Terry raised his voice and began to yell, too.

"Then why did you agree?"

"Because I thought you and I could start a relationship. I figured that if we were together around Sean, you would get over him!" Terry explained.

"I'll never get over him. I love him!" Angela screamed back.

"Good. If that's the way you want it, you can have him. If I see him, I'll tell him where you are and he can come back and get you," Terry said as he started his motorcycle and sped off down the trail leaving Angela standing behind with her mouth hanging open in disbelief.

Thomas stood twenty feet behind Angela.

"What is happening to the young men of today's world?" he asked himself.

They were always leaving their women in the most dangerous, desolate places. If the woman agreed to couple, the men left them. If the woman refused, as this one did, she was still left behind. Thomas made up his mind to give this a lot of thought on a cold night when he became a little bored. It seemed to him that the woman could not win no matter what she did.

He would think about that later. Right now he had work to do. He ran the remaining distance that separated him and the girl and swung his stick as hard as he could. It hit her on the neck and her head went flying into the tall weeds on the opposite side of the trail. Her hands went straight up into the air and seemed to be reaching for the sky as a stream of blood shot out the top of her neck. As quickly as her hands had gone up, they went down to her side again. She fell onto the dirt on her back.

Thomas had no time to admire his work. He heard the whining sound of the motorcycle as it returned. This came as no surprise. Today's men may leave the women, but they always came back for them.

Thomas stepped across the trail and stood in the tall weeds. He looked down and saw Angela's head lying at his feet. He kicked it away from him as he waited for the motorcycle to reach him. He drew his stick back, and at the exact moment Terry passed the trail, he swung it. The stick connected with Terry's chest and knocked him off the motorcycle. Terry landed on the ground and the motorcycle headed down the trail without a rider.

He stepped onto the trail and looked down at Terry. He was not dead yet, but his chest was crushed, and he was struggling to breathe. Thomas stared at him for a full minute until he took his last breath and died. He didn't search the bodies for weapons or anything else. He needed nothing that these interlopers had brought with them from the outside world. He had everything he needed.

CHAPTER 11

"This looks like a good place," Joe Petrie said as he pulled his three-wheeler over, parked it with the front wheel halfway up a small mound, jumped off, and went around the back of it. He turned Nancy around to face him and kissed her deeply.

"What are we going to do here?" she asked as she feigned shyness and surprise that they had stopped on the trail.

"What do you think? Can't you see the way I parked? I gave this a lot of thought, and I have been looking for just the right place," Joe answered.

"What are you talking about?"

"Look," Joe said as he turned her head around. "You see the angle of the three-wheeler? Now, look where you are, and where I'm standing."

"I understand now," Nancy answered. She understood it perfectly. She could lean forward on the seat of the three-wheeler, drop her pants, and Joe could make love to her from behind. That way they would not have to lie on the cold ground or lean against a rough tree.

Joe thought of everything. She guessed that was one of the reasons she had always loved him. She was afraid that once they were married, Joe would lose some of his creative and adventurous spirit. As she pulled down her pants and felt the cold wind rush across her thighs, she knew that would never happen. She leaned as far as she could over the seat and spread her legs slightly.

"You are going to have to do better than that," Joe said as he slipped his hand between her legs and stroked her.

Instinctively she spread her legs apart wider and felt him as he removed his hand and replaced it with something better. She stood on her tiptoes and leaned farther forward so he could penetrate her with all he had. He took long even strokes, and she moaned from the pleasure he was giving her. She knew he was enjoying it too from the sounds he made behind her.

Joe reached around her and put his hand under her jacket. He felt her breasts through her shirt. He wasn't sure if it was because she was aroused or if she was cold, but her nipples were as hard as rocks. He twisted them slightly as he plunged himself into her with more rapid and shorter strokes. After a few minutes he shuddered and let his passion flow into her. He laid his head on her back and closed his eyes.

"Don't move," Nancy pleaded.

"What?"

"Don't move a muscle. I want to feel you inside of me for a little longer. Please just stay right where you are."

That was fine with Joe. He liked the position he was in. After a few moments he felt himself getting aroused again. He waited until he had a full erection before he began making love to her again. He started gradually by taking long, slow strokes as he made love to the woman he had loved for as long as he could remember.

****

Thomas waited and watched as they coupled. He wondered how anything ever got done in the outside world. It seemed, from the people he had come into contact with in the last twenty-four hours, that all they did was couple and fight, or fight over not coupling. He was glad that he lived in the woods where life was not so complicated. For some reason, Thomas did not think the couple he was watching at this moment would fight after they had coupled. They coupled in a different way from the others. They seemed to share a compassion in coupling that consisted of giving mutual pleasure to each other instead of seeking their own gratification. He knew that this man would not leave this woman alone in the woods. He was ready to attack when the man stopped coupling and turned the woman around to face him. The man lifted her legs and she wrapped them around his waist tightly as he entered her again. He continued pounding himself into her as her moans grew louder and louder. When Thomas saw the man's legs began to shake violently he knew now was the time. He raised his stick high and ran out of the woods toward the couple. The woman's eyes were closed and she did not see him standing in front of her.

The man was pounding her with such an intensity that he was oblivious to the world around him and did not hear Thomas stop behind him.

Thomas brought the stick down hard with all of his might and it went through the man's back and pierced through the woman's chest, too. The stick, in its forceful downward movement, stopped only when it penetrated the cushion of the three-wheeler's seat and hit the metal.

There were no screams from the man, or the woman. They had died instantly. Thomas pulled his stick from their bodies, and they stayed in the same position. Their lips were barely touching, and their bodies were still connected.

A single tear fell gently down Nancy's face and mingled on their lips. They had died as they had promised each other to live. Together as one, forever.

****

Arthur followed Sean and J.P. up one trail and down another. He could tell that they were holding back waiting for him. He knew that if it weren't for him, they would be going twice as fast as they were. They topped one hill and rode down to the bottom of it and stopped. The area in front of them was cleared of trees and was full of deep pits.

"This must be where they threw the grenades," Sean said.

"Then there has to be a concrete bunker around here somewhere," J.P. added.

"There are more than likely several of them," Arthur agreed.

"Let's go," Sean said. "Let's ride the side of the pits."

They all took off and rode up the wall of the pits. Arthur was shocked that he did it so well the first time he tried it. He went faster and faster around the side. As he looked down, he hit a muddy spot and slammed into the wall of the pit and slid down to the bottom of it. He landed hard as the breath was knocked out of him.

"Are you all right, Dad?" Sean asked as he drove next to him.

"Yes," Arthur wheezed.

"Good. I would hate to go home and tell Mom that I got my old man killed."

"I would hate to have to put you through that, too. That would be awfully selfish of me," Arthur said sarcastically.

"Next time you fall on the side of a hill like that, lean toward the wall and you'll just slide down without hurting yourself," Sean suggested.

"I'll try and remember that."

"Are you ready to ride?" J.P. asked.

"I've got a better idea," Arthur said. "Why don't you two take off and go riding by yourself. I'll stay here and play in the pits. I need the practice anyway."

"Are you sure?" they asked.

"Positive. You two go on. You can swing back by here in a little while," Arthur answered.

Arthur saw that Sean had a concerned look on his face, but he reluctantly agreed to the suggestion.

"Okay. We'll be back in an hour."

Arthur knew that Sean would not get an opportunity to ride his motorcycle in such a great place again for quite a while. He wanted him to take full advantage of it while he could. He watched as Sean and J.P. rode out of the pit and up the side of a steep hill. They would have never tried that hill if he were following them. They were already driving twice as fast over rough terrain than they had all day while he was following them. It could have been pitch dark outside and they would not have had to worry about seeing where they were going. The broad smiles on their faces as they raced away would have given them enough light to see.

Arthur played on the hills for a while until the rain began falling harder and his tires got very little, if any, traction on the sides of the pit. He drove out and took a small trail that led around the steep hill that Sean and J.P. had climbed. He reasoned that they would meet up somewhere on the top.

****

Damuth Hendricks and Gerard Bradley stopped the

110

motorcycle as they pulled inside the bunker. It was a three sided structure made of concrete. It was eight feet high and had a concrete roof. Damuth tried to impress Gerard with his knowledge of military maneuvers and procedures.

"They would stand here and throw the grenades over the bunker," Damuth said as he pointed to the roof. "If the grenade didn't go far enough and landed on this side of that hill, the concrete roof would protect them as they ran back inside the bunker."

Gerard tried to act interested, but he wasn't. He was just glad they had found a place to get out of the cold rain. He was freezing and felt a cold coming on.

"Why don't we build a fire? I'm cold," Gerard said.

"We could if we had any dry wood," Damuth answered.

"What about those pine branches over there?"

Damuth looked where Gerard was pointing at the end of the bunker. He saw a pile of pine limbs that seemed to be out of place. It didn't look as if the wind had blown them underneath the bunker. They were stacked too neatly.

"I guess they will work, if they're dry."

"They're dry," Gerard said as he pulled a large branch from the stack and placed it on the floor of the bunker and lit it.

The pine needles caught fire instantly and burned quickly.

"Get another branch before this one goes out," Gerard said.

Damuth pulled on a large branch that was stubborn. It was entangled with several more. He jerked harder and it finally broke free and he lost his balance and fell. He looked up as the other branches fell to the floor.

"What is that?" he asked as he looked through the space where the branches had been.

"It looks like a truck," Gerard said as he helped Damuth up.

They walked over and moved some of the other branches out of the way until they could plainly see a Ford pickup truck.

"Who would hide a truck here?" Damuth asked.

"It's probably stolen. Maybe the people who stole it are going to come back later and take whatever parts they need off of it," Gerard said.

"You're probably right. I don't want to be here when they come back," Damuth added.

"Me neither. Let's get out of here," Gerard said with urgency.

"Wait a minute. I want to look inside of it," Damuth said.

"This is no time to be macho. Let's go," Gerard urged.

"We will. The people who stole this truck won't be back until later, when it's dark, or else they would be here now," Damuth argued.

"I don't really want to take any chances on that."

"It will only take a minute. You can wait here if you like," Damuth said as he walked over and looked inside the truck.

He stepped back quickly.

"There's blood all over the seat and the hood! Lots of blood! Whoever was in that truck is dead after losing all that blood. The windshield is broken, but I don't think this truck has been in a wreck," Damuth said in horror.

"I don't care what happened! Let's go, now!" Gerard said as he fidgeted nervously and moved his feet up and down as if he were walking, but he stayed in the same spot.

"You're right. Let's go. We have to tell someone about this," Damuth stated with determination.

As they turned back toward their bikes, they stood face to face with a tall man who wore an old hat and carried a big stick. They huddled together as he walked toward them.

"I can't let you tell anyone about that truck," Thomas said softly.

"We won't tell anyone. We promise," Damuth said.

"I know you won't. I thought I hid it pretty well. Who would have thought a couple of nosy sissies like you two would have found it?"

"We're not sissies," Gerard protested.

"Don't argue with him," Damuth said under his breath. "We don't want to piss him off."

"It's too late for that. I was pissed off the first time I laid eyes on you," Thomas answered.

"There are two of us," Gerard said.

"I know. I can count, not too high, mind you, but I can count."

"We don't want to hurt you. So if you will please stand aside and get out of our way, everything will be fine," Damuth stated.

Thomas laughed loudly and grabbed Damuth by the throat and squeezed. Gerard began to pound Thomas with blows that he did not feel as they bounced off him. He picked Damuth up until his feet no longer touched the ground as he tightened the grip he had on his throat. Damuth's feet swung wildly in the air as his hands tried to free his throat from the grasp that was taking his breath. Not much time passed before his legs ceased flailing and his hands hung limply at his side. Thomas dropped his body to the floor of the bunker. It landed with a sickening thud.

"You killed him!" Gerard screamed as he dropped to his knees and cradled Damuth's head in his arms.

Thomas covered Gerard's face with his huge hand and pushed him to the floor. He gripped the face harder and slammed the back of Gerard's head over and over again onto the concrete floor until the area around Gerard's head was red.

Thomas released his grip on Gerard's face and stepped away. The two men lying on the floor had surprised him by fighting back. He had expected them to run instead. Their blood returning to the earth would produce something useful he thought as he walked back into the woods in search of the other motorcycle riders.

There were only a few hours left until dark, and the aches in his body told him that he needed to rest tonight. He needed to sit by the fire and feel the warmth on his sore muscles. He needed to sit quietly and hear the sounds of the night that emanated from his woods. He had not slept at all last night, and fatigue was coming over him quickly. The last twenty-four hours had taxed his strength tremendously. What he wanted came last. Protecting the forest and its inhabitants would always be his first priority for as long as he lived.

Besides, Thomas remembered that he had a guest waiting for him at his bunker. James Foster. It would not be polite to keep him waiting for dinner too long. Thomas smiled as he thought about James. Thomas would insist that James stay for dinner. Of course he would have to agree. He would stay no matter how much he protested. He had to stay. James Foster was going to be the dinner for tonight.

CHAPTER 12

Mark and Tiffanie exited the woods and came upon a small trail that they followed for several miles before he stopped.

"Are we lost?" Tiffanie asked.

"I'm afraid so. I just knew I shouldn't have cut through those trees that didn't have any sign of a trail."

"I'm not going to argue with that," Tiffanie said as she pulled the briars and pine needles from her hair.

The ride through the thick woods and underbrush had been rough on both of them. Their faces were full of scratches, and Mark had already pulled three ticks from his neck. He was relieved when they had finally gotten through the woods and found this trail. At least someone had used it recently. He saw the tread marks of a motorcycle in the mud.

"We'll be able to get out of here in a little while," Mark said as he tried to reassure Tiffanie. He hoped that he could reassure himself, too.

"Are you sure?"

"Of course, I'm sure. You see those tire tracks. They are not filled with rainwater yet. That means that someone rode past here in about the last hour," Mark answered.

"And just how did you put a time frame on that observation?" Tiffanie asked jokingly.

"By the density of the ground multiplied by the rate the rain is falling."

"Bullshit."

"I know, but it sure sounded intelligent, didn't it?" Mark asked.

"You should have been a scout for the Calvary."

"No way," Mark replied. "They rode horses, not motorcycles. Besides they fought savage Indians. The only thing I have to fight out here are ticks and a few mosquitoes that are too stupid to know that they are not supposed to bite in the cold."

"There are enough of all of them," Tiffanie said as she swatted at a cloud of mosquitoes that swarmed around her head.

"You won't be bothered by them much longer. As fast as the temperature is dropping, they will not be a problem for much longer."

"For some reason, that doesn't make me feel any better," she answered.

"Do you want to rest here a while?" Mark asked.

"Hell no! Let's get back to the truck as fast as we can. I'm dying for a Coke and some of those sandwiches we brought," Tiffanie answered.

"Is eating all you think about?"

"Lately it is. But I have a reason."

"What reason?" he asked.

"I'm eating for two."

"Two what?"

"Two people, you idiot."

Tiffanie was glad that she had finally told him. She had hoped all day that a chance would come when she could unburden herself of the secret she had carried inside of her for over a month.

Mark stopped the motorcycle and turned off the key and looked back at her.

"You want to explain that?" Mark inquired.

"Do I have to spell it out for you?"

"No. Just tell me nice and slow."

"I'm pregnant."

"Pregnant?"

"Yes. I am P R E G N A ....." Tiffanie answered as she began to spell the word.

"But are you sure?" Mark interrupted.

"I'm positive. I even went to the doctor."

"How could that happen?" Mark tried to ask innocently.

"Do I have to tell you that, too?" Tiffanie wondered.

"You know what I mean. I thought you were on the pill."

"I was, Mark. But does an aspirin get rid of your headache every time you take one?"

"No, but I thought the pill was sure fire."

"It usually is. You are always telling me that I am one in a million. I guess this proves you right," Tiffanie said lovingly.

116

There was a long silence between them as Mark contemplated what Tiffanie had told him.

"Are you angry with me?" she finally broke the stillness and asked him.

"No, I'm not. What are you going to do about it?"

"I don't want to have an abortion, and I'm not going to, either," Tiffanie declared.

"I would never ask you to do that," Mark argued.

"I know you wouldn't. I just wanted to let my feelings be known up front."

There was another silence.

"What are **your** feelings?" Tiffanie asked him.

"About what?"

"About the baby."

"I like babies. Of course, I've never had one before. I was even a baby once myself, but I don't remember much about that time," Mark spoke quickly.

Tiffanie pinched his shoulder hard. "I'm serious. What do you want to do about it?"

"I guess we'll have to get married," Mark said quickly.

"We don't have to do anything. If you want to get married, we will. But we will do it because we want to, not because we have to."

"Are you going to be a nag like this and pick at every little thing I say after we get married?" Mark asked.

"Probably."

"Okay. I accept your proposal. I'll marry you. But there are two things we have to get straight right here and now," Mark answered.

"Such as?"

"If it's a boy, he will be able to ride motorcycles with me. We have to clear that up right now."

"I guess I could agree to that. What's the other thing?" Tiffanie asked.

"If it's a girl, she will be able to ride motorcycles with me."

"Only if I can come along," Tiffanie responded.

"It's a deal. When can we get married?" Mark asked.

"Why don't we talk about that after you get me out of these woods," Tiffanie answered as she swatted at another mosquito.

"I'll do that. Daddy Mark will save his kid and soon to be fat wife from the dreaded horde of mosquitoes."

Mark started the motorcycle engine and pressed the shift lever into first gear. He was ready to take off when he turned to Tiffanie again.

"Is it safe for you to be riding motorcycles in your condition?"

"This will be my last trip."

Thomas almost screamed out in agreement with her as he rushed from the stand of trees through which they had emerged and held his stick high, ready to attack. He had been following them through the woods for over a mile. While they were fighting each low hanging branch, he was walking easily through the clear parts. He knew his forest and moved with ease through it. He had not had any trouble keeping up with them. In fact, he could have killed them when they first stopped and started talking, if he had wanted to do that. But he didn't. He had misjudged these two young people. He assumed that they would couple as the others had. Then he could kill them effortlessly while they were preoccupied. When he realized that they were going to leave without coupling, he had not moved fast enough to reach them. He was a split second too late. Mark let the clutch out on the motorcycle just as Thomas swung his stick and went tumbling to the ground from the force that he had put behind the thrust.

Thomas got to his feet and went back into the woods. He would catch them on the other side of this stand of trees. They would be trying to reach the last three remaining riders. If he had his way, they would never achieve that goal.

Mark and Tiffanie rode down the trail without looking back. They never knew how close to them death had come. They raced down the trail at top speed until Mark saw the motorcycle lying in his path. He stopped beside it. Tiffanie started screaming immediately. He had to stifle a scream too as he saw the body of Terry Richardson lying twenty feet ahead of him.

Mark stopped his motorcycle and knelt beside the body. There was no doubt in his mind that Terry was dead.

"What happened? Did he have a wreck?" Tiffanie asked as she controlled her fear.

"I don't think so. There's nothing in the trail he could have hit that could have caved in his chest like this," Mark answered as he looked around him.

"Let's get out of here!" Tiffanie said. She was shaking violently and felt as if she were going to be sick. She forced the bile that rose in her throat back down to her stomach.

"Wait a minute. Where's Angela? She was riding with him."

Tiffanie screamed in answer to his question and pointed to the body lying on the trail a few away. They both knew it was Angela even though her head was missing. Her figure was rather unique.

Tiffanie could not stop herself from throwing up as she stared at the body. She got off the motorcycle and threw up what was in her stomach from breakfast and continued heaving without throwing up any solid matter long after her breakfast was gone. Mark tried to comfort her and calm her down. It took several minutes to accomplish that enough to put her back on the motorcycle and head down the trail again.

Thomas emerged from the woods too late again. He shook his fist angrily and cursed at them as they drove away. This time Tiffanie and Mark did see him.

****

Sean and J.P. rode up and down every hill that came into their path. They took every jump off every mound that got in their way. They were having the time of their lives and did not let the cold, drizzling rain that had started falling again bother them. They had come to Camp Leder to ride and enjoy life, and that's what they were doing. They lost all track of time and the world around them as they climbed the steepest hill they had come to yet and took it with pride and the spirit of adventure.

Mark followed the trail until it came to the main dirt road. He knew exactly where he was now. Sean, Mr. Billings, and J.P. had taken the first trail and all the others had gone to different trails to the left. The truck was to the right. If the others were still alive, they had no idea of the danger that was lurking in the woods waiting for them. If they were dead, like Terry and Angela were, he could not do anything to help them anyway. His mind was filled with much indecision as he pondered his choices. Tiffanie sobbed loudly as he sat there and made up his mind. He turned to the right and drove over and parked the motorcycle next to the truck and they got off of it. He opened the truck door, climbed in and started it up as Tiffanie got in on the passenger side and locked the door behind her.

"Let's go!" she screamed as he sat there with the motor idling.

"I can't," he said.

"What's the matter? Is there something wrong with the truck?"

"No. I just can't leave the others out there. I have to warn them," Mark answered as he got out of the truck.

"You can't! That crazy man will kill us!" Tiffanie screamed through her tears.

"Not us. Maybe me. You are going to get the police while I warn the others," Mark replied.

"I can't leave you out here alone. I'll go with you."

"No, you won't. You'll do exactly as I say. Those are my friends out there. One of them is like a father to me. I can't leave them to be killed by that butcher. Didn't you see what he did to Angela?"

"Yes," Tiffanie said as the thought made her swallow another lump of something that came into her throat.

"We're wasting time. Do you know how to get out of here?"

"I think so," Tiffanie said slowly.

"Don't think, Tiffanie. Be sure."

"Yes. I take a right at the end of this road, then a left when I reach the main highway."

"That's right. Now get out of here, and be careful."

"I will," Tiffanie said as she slid behind the wheel and pulled the shift into reverse and backed up. She slammed on the brakes and let the sliding of the wheels move the back of the truck around until it was facing the road.

Mark ran to his motorcycle and cranked it up. As usual, it started the first time. He looked at Tiffanie the second before she drove away and mouthed the words slowly so she would be sure to understand.

"I love you."

Then he sped away in the same direction the others had gone.

****

Thomas waited at the end of the trail. The motorcycle and its passengers should have been here by now. They would have had to come this way to get to the others. They were long overdue. Then it dawned on him that they may not try to warn the others. They may just try to save themselves.

"Of course, that's just what they did," he mumbled.

The campsite was in the other direction. If they went there, they could get away and bring back the police. It didn't bother Thomas too much about the police. He could hide from them forever. But it did bother him that they might get away after violating his woods. And he could not get the others with police crawling all over the place. He ran back into the woods toward the campsite. He knew of a shortcut, but he doubted that it would save enough time to reach them before they left. He had barely gone into the woods when he heard the whine of the motorcycle as it passed ten feet from him. It was the same man that he had seen before, only this time, the woman was not with him. The man had sent her for help so he could warn his friends.

"Very noble of him," Thomas said softly. "I think I will kill him quickly."

****

Tiffanie floored the truck and made the first turn on two wheels as she drove as fast as she could to get help. She prayed as she drove that it would not be too late when that help came back for Mark and any of the others that might still be alive right now.

The rain began falling harder and the drops began to freeze on her windshield forming tiny icicles. The windshield wipers did nothing to clear the windshield. It only smeared the ice around and obstructed her vision more. She strained her eyes to see through the spaces where ice had not yet formed. She turned the heater on defrost all the way up, but it was slow in melting the ice. The second turn was upon her before she realized it and she slammed on the brakes. The water mixed with a thin layer of ice on the road made the truck go into a skid as she fought the steering wheel. She lost the battle as the truck slid off the road and into a ravine.

****

Mark didn't slow down as he passed the bodies of Joe and Nancy Petrie. There was no help he could give them. He surprised himself when he didn't even shed a tear for two people who had been lifelong friends. He knew the time for grief would be later, after he warned the living, if there were any living people left in the world. He felt at this moment as if he were the only living person on this earth, The only one except for the old man with the big stick.

****

Arthur rode the trails for a while before he came back to the pit where he had started. He was pretty proud of himself. He had practiced jumping the smaller mounds and riding on the rear wheel. He was still not nearly as good as J.P. and Sean, but he didn't harbor that hope anyway.

The rain fell on his face and he thought about something J.P. had said earlier. If the pit was caused by grenades, there had to be a bunker nearby. Arthur wiped the rain from his face and knew it would be dry in that bunker. He could get out of the freezing wind, too.

He rode up the small hill and through a stretch of tall weeds. Then he spotted it. It was like a friendly port on a stormy sea. The gray concrete wall beckoned to him to come in and share the warmth and safety. The bunker was straight ahead. Someone else must have gotten the same idea, he thought as he saw the thin waft of smoke coming from it. He revved up the engine and rode on the rear wheel to the bunker.

He saw the bodies of Damuth and Gerard immediately as he drove into the bunker.

He looked around quickly for any other bodies while he prayed that if there were, Sean would not be one of them. He was relieved when he didn't see any more bodies. He also felt a twinge of guilt for being glad that it was Damuth and Gerard, and not Sean. They deserved to live, too.

Arthur left the bunker much faster than he had ridden into it. He had one thought on his mind. He had to find Sean, J.P., Mark and any of the others. He stopped at the top of the steep hill that he had been afraid to try earlier. He climbed it without even thinking. What if Sean and J.P. came back looking for him? He tried to remember how long ago they had left. He couldn't. His mind was boggled from worry, and he couldn't think clearly. But, surely, it had to be over an hour ago. If they came back looking for him and he wasn't here, they might wait for him and fall into the same trap that Damuth and Gerard had fallen into. But what if they were in danger at this very moment? He would have to warn them before it was too late. Arthur felt the rain falling on him as he sat there contemplating his next move. His mind was so engrossed that he did not feel the cold. A few moments ago he had thought he would freeze to death. Now, he was sweating profusely from worry.

Arthur revved his motor again. He could not sit idly by while there were people in danger. He climbed the next hill and barely made it to the top. He had driven fifty feet when he heard the sound of the motorcycle coming toward him. The rain fell in sheets as he stared at the rider. It was Mark.

"Arthur, thank God you are all right. You won't believe what's going on," Mark said as he pulled up beside him.

"Don't bet any money on it," Arthur answered.

"They are all dead!" Mark blurted out.

"What about Sean and J.P. ?"

"I don't know. That's why I'm up here. I came looking for all of you," Mark told Arthur.

"What about Tiffanie?" Arthur asked with concern.

"She's all right. I sent her back to that small town in the truck to get the police."

"Good. Why didn't you go with her?" Arthur wondered.

"I had to warn all of you, at least all that's left alive."

"Who else is dead?" Arthur asked. He was surprised that he could ask such a question so calmly.

"What do you mean, who else?"

"I found Damuth and Gerard down below in a bunker. Who did you find?"

Mark took a deep breath and let it out slowly. They both acted as if they were trading talk about something else besides dead people. He decided not to mention it. Time was slipping by, and they still did not know anything about J.P. or Sean.

"I found Terry and Angela on one of the trails. Her head was missing, but I'm pretty sure it was her. Joe and Nancy are dead, too."

"That means that you, me, Sean and J.P. are the only ones left," Arthur said.

"We can't be sure about them."

"Let's go find them," Arthur said as he started his bike and backed it up and headed it in the same direction that Mark was facing.

"Do we split up? We would have a better chance of finding them faster," Mark said.

"I don't think that would be a good idea. We would also have a better chance of getting killed. There is safety in numbers, even though it didn't help the others."

"I don't know about safety, but I do know there is a certain amount of comfort in having company. I was beginning to think that I was the only person alive except for that old man."

"What old man?" Arthur asked.

"I didn't tell you about him? My God, I must be losing my mind! I think he is the one doing all the killing. He ran after me and Tiffanie with a stick about eight feet long. It looked more like a limb. I couldn't be sure, but I think he would have crushed our heads in with it."

"He may be responsible. I don't know, but one thing I do know is that if we meet anyone in these woods that we don't know and they get in our way, we're going to take them out," Arthur answered.

"There's no one left in these woods that we know, not alive anyway."

Arthur saw no need to reply to Mark's last remark. The reality was too painful to think about. He also felt sorry for the ones who had died. Even Angela. He may not have thought she was right for Sean, but he didn't hate her enough to wish she were dead. Arthur tried not to think about Terry. He didn't care for him at all, and he found it hard to find any sympathy in his heart for him. Arthur liked Damuth and he hardly knew Gerard, but he seemed like he was a nice enough guy. And Joe and Nancy. They died before they even had a chance to live. They were perfect for each other. They were like rare diamonds in a pile of black coal. They shined and brightened everyone, everywhere they went. As Arthur thought about them, he wished that he could kill the man who had killed them. Arthur also felt another emotion besides revenge coming over him. That emotion was fear. He was afraid for Sean, J.P., and Mark. He was also afraid for himself. He didn't want to die either.

****

J.P. stopped his motorcycle next to Sean's and lit a cigarette. He inhaled deeply and blew the smoke out slowly.

"You think it's about time we headed back?" he asked Sean.

"Yes, I guess it is time we checked on the old man."

"He's not so old," J.P. argued.

"I know, but he might be if he crashes his face into the side of too many more hills."

"Nah. I think it will just make him tougher," J.P. answered.

"Damn. Then we had better get back and check up on him. If he gets any tougher than he is, I don't think I could stand it," Sean said.

Sean and J.P. drove up the steep hill and headed back to the area where they had left Arthur to practice his riding. They unknowingly took a wrong turn at the end of the trail and drove in the opposite direction from the pit.

****

Arthur and Mark drove down several trails looking for Sean and J.P. before they finally stopped at the end of one. The wind had begun to blow harder and made a loud eerie sound as it rushed through the trees.

"I don't know where the hell they went!" Arthur shouted so Mark could hear him over the engines of the motorcycles and the howling wind.

"Do you think they went back to the campsite?"

"No. There is no way Sean and J.P. could leave me alone out here any more than you could," Arthur shouted. "Just in case I don't get a chance to tell you later, Mark, I appreciate you coming back to warn us. That's the bravest thing I've ever seen in my life."

"I have to tell you, I don't feel very brave. I'm scared to death," Mark replied.

"Don't feel bad about that. You are not alone."

"What do we do now?" Mark asked. "Do we keep searching the other trails? They could be almost anywhere."

Arthur looked around him. Mark was right. The way the wind was blowing the rain sideways, they could pass within twenty feet of Sean and J.P. and not see them. He looked above him and could barely see the top of the steep hill as the rain slacked off.

"Up there," Arthur pointed. "If we could get up there, we might be able to spot them."

"I'm ready when you are," Mark said in a hurry.

Arthur took the lead and began climbing the hill first. The

street tire on the back of his motorcycle began spinning rapidly and he slid backwards down the hill. He remembered what Sean had said and shifted his body weight to the right and leaned into the side of the hill. He slid down and was still sitting on his motorcycle when he landed on the bottom.

"I'll go. You wait here. Those tires will never be able to take that hill in this mud," Mark said.

"The hell they won't. I'll get up there even if I have to carry this son-of-a-bitch on my back," Arthur said as he revved his engine and rode up the hill again.

This time he went at a slight angle instead of trying to go straight up. The tires began spinning again as he dug into the mud. He didn't bother to try and shift his weight this time. It would not have done any good. The angle he was climbing the hill made it impossible to lean. If he fell this time, the motorcycle would fall on him and crush him when he hit the bottom of the hill. He eased back on the throttle and reduced his speed. The rear tire stopped spinning as fast as it had before, but it was still not getting much traction and began slipping. Arthur decided there was only one thing to do. He gave it all the gas he could and leaned forward to try and take some of the weight off the rear tire. That helped a little, but he felt the tire sliding again. He held on and actually tried pushing his body forward in a motion that looked as if he were trying to scoot the motorcycle up the hill. The rear tire stopped spinning when it hit an old tree that had died and began to rot near the top of the hill. The rotted wood gave the tire enough traction to top the hill. It took Arthur forty feet before he could bring his motorcycle to a complete stop. His brakes were almost completely gone now.

Mark revved his engine and, with his big mud tires and powerful engine, had no trouble making it to the top of the hill.

"You did great, Arthur. Sean and J.P. would be proud of you."

"Let's hope we live long enough to tell them," Arthur prayed.

Arthur and Mark looked around the top of the hill. It was like a small plateau on the opposite side from where they had ridden up. There was a dropoff that went straight down. They could see the tops of huge pine trees.

"We can't go down that way, and I don't see them," Mark said.

"Me, neither," Arthur said with a heavy sadness in his voice.

"That doesn't mean anything. They could be waiting until the rain stops. You know how cold natured J.P. is. He's so skinny that he gets cold easily. He doesn't have enough body fat to keep him warm."

"Maybe you're right," Arthur agreed with Mark, but he didn't believe it.

"Let's go back down the hill and look for them again. See, the rain is almost stopped now. They'll probably be waiting for us at the pit where they left you."

Arthur drove his motorcycle to the side they had come up. Mark joined him and looked down.

"It looks a lot steeper from up here, doesn't it?" Mark observed.

"Sure does. I hope these street tires can get me back down."

"You can ride down with me." Mark suggested. "We can always come back for your motorcycle."

"Thanks, but no. If Sean is dead, this motorcycle is all that I have left to remember him by. Besides that, if I ever get away from these woods, I don't think I will ever be coming back."

"I'll go along with that," Mark sadly agreed.

"Are you ready?" Arthur asked.

"Wait a minute. I can try to ride it down for you. I've been riding a long time. I think I can handle it a little better than you can," Mark offered.

The wind calmed and the rain stopped completely as Arthur looked down the steep side of the hill. It was as if the weather had joined with the woods in some form of evil pact to lull him into a false sense of security. It was as if the trees themselves were beckoning to him to drive down the hill any way he wanted to. They would take care of him. Arthur surveyed the hillside with his eyes. He did not trust the trees, nor the wind that pretended it was asleep only to rise and blow him away from the hillside and carry him to his death. He spotted a small strip of land going down the hill that looked to have more branches lying on the ground than other places did. The branches would help him to maintain traction. That may have solved one problem. There was nothing on the side of the hill that would solve the other one, his brakes. Or should he say the absence of his brakes. His only hope would be to put the engine in first gear and hope that it would slow him enough to control the motorcycle on the trip down.

Arthur looked at Mark and nodded his head in a signal that he was ready. The second before he was ready to start down the hill, he heard the sound behind him.

Arthur looked at Mark. He had heard it, too. They looked around and saw Thomas holding his big stick firmly in his hand. He made no movement toward them. As he and Arthur looked into each other's eyes, it was like a contract had been made between them without saying a word. It was a contract of life, or death. A contract that would be carried out in the next few minutes.

"What now? That's the guy I saw on the trail," Mark said.

"I figured that. You go down the hill. I'm going to take care of him."

"How?"

"He's standing at the edge of the cliff. If I can slide into him, or scare him enough, he may panic and get careless and lose his footing and fall over the cliff," Arthur answered.

"I don't think you'll scare him into jumping off that cliff," Mark warned.

"Then I'll push his ass off and send him to Hell."

"What if he moves away, or you can't stop?" Mark could only worry for Arthur.

"Then I'll go off the cliff and wait for him in Hell. Then I'll hunt him down and drag him through every single fire when he gets there," Arthur stated in a frenzy.

"This is crazy. Why don't we just go down the hill and find Sean and J.P.?"

"Because of what you said earlier. You were right. Sean and J.P. would not leave me out here alone for as long as they did. They would have come back for me if they could, but they didn't. That can mean only one thing. They were not able to come back for me because he killed them, or left them hurt somewhere," Arthur explained.

"It could be like we agreed. They could have been waiting for the rain to stop. You remember, J.P. doesn't have any body fat."

"That's what you said,Mark. Now, do what I tell you to do. Get ready to ride down the side of that hill. Save yourself. Sean and J.P. are gone."

"Please come with me," Mark pleaded.

"Sorry son. I've got something to do right now," Arthur said as he revved his engine up all the way.

Mark did not try to argue anymore. The look on Arthur's face told him it would be useless.

"Thanks for coming back," Arthur shouted to Mark as he released the clutch lever and the motorcycle went speeding off in the direction of the old man standing at the edge of the cliff.

Mark watched in horror as Arthur rode across the top of the hill. At the speed Arthur was traveling, it only took a few seconds to cover the distance between him and the old man. Mark could tell that Arthur never released the pressure on the throttle as he drove toward the old man.

The man took a quick step to the side, but Arthur laid the motorcycle on its side and spun the rear tire around and knocked the old man over the edge as he and his motorcycle went hurtling over the cliff, too.

Mark got off his motorcycle and ran to the edge of the cliff. He saw the broken tree branches where Arthur had fallen, but he couldn't see Arthur or the motorcycle. The cliff was too high, and the rain and wind had started raging again with the same ferocity and intensity that it had displayed earlier.

Mark saw no sign of the old man, either. Arthur had kept his promise. He had sent the old man to Hell. Mark said a silent prayer and prayed that Arthur had not gone to Hell with him. He wiped the rain from his face, but his eyes filled up with more water as soon as he had dried them. It puddled up and ran down his face. He didn't wipe the water away this time. The water in his eyes was tears, not rain. The tears that flowed from his eyes would make a larger puddle than all the rain that had fallen in these woods today.

He returned to his motorcycle and rode carefully down the side of the hill. The danger was gone, there was no need to hurry. He would go back to the campsite and wait. Tiffanie would be back soon with the police. Then he could begin to put this horrible ordeal behind him. He said another silent prayer for God to give him the strength he would need to eventually be able do that.

****

As soon as the noise of the motorcycle faded as it went down the other side of the hill, a hand appeared on the top of the cliff. Thomas had begun to worry if he would have had to hang on to the ledge much longer. If he had let go, he would be at the bottom with the man who pushed him over the edge. He would be dead, too. He had been lucky. He had been able to grab hold of a jagged rock that jutted out just below the top as he fell. The young man standing above him could not see him as he hung on for his life.

Thomas pulled himself up onto the top and rested until he caught his breath. These people were crazy, he thought to himself. If they weren't coupling and fighting among themselves, they were trying to kill him by pushing him off a cliff. These people did not even care if they died.

"Three more to go," he said as he stood up and walked through a row of bushes. There was a long, winding trail that led to the bottom of the hill. Thomas had used this trail many times. It was the one he had used to beat Arthur and Mark to the top a few minutes earlier. He knew that he would come out at the bottom of the hill on the other side.

CHAPTER 13

The wind blew the cold rain through the crack in the driver's side window and landed on Tiffanie's face and woke her up. She opened her eyes slowly. She was lying on the passenger side of the truck where she had been thrown as the truck slid into the ditch. The memory of what happened came rushing over her. How long had she been knocked out? There was no way of knowing the answer to that question. She was not wearing a watch. Tiffanie did know one thing, she had to get help. She tried to rise up, but a splitting pain filled her head. She closed her eyes and laid her head back down.

"The pain will stop in a minute," she told herself.

The pain did not subside as she hoped it would. She must have hit her head in the accident, she thought. That made no difference. She had to get to the police and save Mark and the others. Her pain was nothing compared to what they might be experiencing at this very moment.

She rose up again and the pain in her head was worse this time. It was accompanied by dizziness and blurred vision. She strained her eyes to look around the truck. The sight that greeted her made her cringe. The floor of the truck was quickly filling with the water from the ditch. There was no doubt in her mind that it would consume her soon if she did not get out of the truck.

She amassed all the strength within her as she tried to rise up again. This time she managed to sit upright. She reached for the steering wheel to pull herself up as she looked outside. The main road was just ahead. If she could get to it, she might be able to flag down a passing car. There was still hope to save Mark and any of the others that were still alive.

As she grabbed the door handle, the darkness of unconsciousness overcame her, and she fell back onto the seat again. Her last thoughts as she fought to stay awake were of Mark and the baby she carried inside of her. Mark had shown such happiness when she had told him about the baby. His face was also filled with concern and worry, but that was good. That meant he really did care. He would have made a good father.

None of that made any difference now. Mark was probably dead, and in a few minutes when the truck filled with water she and the baby would die, too. There was nothing that could change that. She and Mark would not know the joy of being parents and spending a lifetime together.

Tiffanie quit fighting. All was lost. She let the blackness that surrounded her pull her into it.

****

Mark reached the bottom of the hill and did not slow down. His patience was gone. He was in a hurry to get out of these woods now. His tires slid as he made a sharp turn and rode toward the campsite. He was passing the grenade pit when he heard the sounds of the other motorcycles coming over the mound. It was Sean and J.P.. He slammed on his brakes and stopped.

"Where's Dad?" Sean asked as he pulled up and stopped in front of Mark.

J.P. stopped next to Sean.

"He's dead!" Mark screamed.

"What do you mean, he's dead?"

Mark thought a moment before he answered. How could he tell them about what he had seen today? Where did he begin? What words could he possibly use to describe the horror of senseless killing?

"Everyone is dead, except us and Tiffanie," Mark finally said.

"Tell me what's going on!" Sean demanded. "And make it quick!"

Mark did his best to relate the events of the day to them. In his excitement he got things out of order, but he did not try to correct it. He doubted if Sean would have the patience to listen anyway. When he got to the part about Arthur, Sean's eyes began to fill with tears that he let flow undaunted down his face.

"And that's it. I ran into you two after that," Mark said as he finished telling his story.

"Show me where Dad is!" Sean screamed.

"It's over the big hill over there," Mark said as he pointed.

"We've got to get to him. He may be not be dead. Maybe he's just hurt."

"No, Sean. He's dead. There is no way on earth that he could have survived that fall. It was at least a two hundred and fifty foot drop straight down. I'm sorry, you just don't know how sorry I am. I loved him like a father, too. But you have to face the fact that he is dead."

Sean stared at Mark. Maybe he and Arthur were playing a joke on him. Maybe they concocted this whole story together just as a prank. Arthur was always playing jokes on him. Like the time Arthur disconnected the battery cables when he had a big night out planned. Or the time Arthur hid in the closet in his bedroom and jumped out and scared him after they had watched a scary movie together. He quickly pushed that thought from his mind. His dad would never be so cruel as to play a sordid joke like this on him. His grief turned to anger as the reality of what Mark had told him sank into his mind.

"You don't seem too upset about it!" he yelled at Mark.

"I've seen so much today that I don't think anything will ever upset me again. Later on tonight, when we get out of these damn woods, I'm going to get angry. I'll probably beat my fists on a wall for an hour. I'll scream at the top of my lungs and try to force the memory of every dead body I've seen today out of my head. But I'll have to wait until later to do that. Right now all I care about is getting out of here," Mark answered Sean.

"Show me where he went off the cliff. I want to go to him."

"It won't do any good."

"Show me anyway!" Sean then demanded.

J.P. had been strangely silent during the time Mark was telling his story. He had listened quietly and patiently. That was his nature, even in the most dire situation. He liked to have all the facts so he could calmly and rationally make his determination about what to do. It did not work this time. This was not a normal situation. It was unlike any situation he had ever been in before, and one that he hoped he would never be in again.

He was filled with many different emotions, including

sadness and anger, and a sense of loss from which he knew he would never completely recover. His mind flashed back to a year ago. He had just moved from a small town to the area where Sean lived to get a better job. He did not know anybody that he could consider a friend before he met Sean. They had become friends immediately. Sean had introduced him to his friends, and he fit in with the crowd perfectly. He was not lonesome anymore. He felt like he belonged again. The fact that Sean's parents were such nice people was an added benefit. J.P.'s own parents still lived in the small town he had moved from, and he didn't see them much. He called them every two weeks and went back home every month or so. Arthur and Elizabeth filled a void in his life that he didn't even know was there until he met them. Elizabeth was like a second mother to him. She talked to him about things that only his own mother could understand.

Arthur was also important in his life. Arthur was a complicated man that did his best to appear uncomplicated. J.P. also knew that Arthur hid his feelings often. Like the night that Sean had moved out to his own place. J.P. remembered it vividly. It was Halloween night, and also Arthur's birthday. He was sitting in a chair in the driveway giving out candy to the neighborhood kid's trick-or-treating as Sean loaded up the last of his belongings from the house. Arthur had shaken Sean's hand firmly and told him he was welcome to move back if things did not work out. J.P. almost smiled at the memory of Arthur trying so hard to be strong as he watched his son drive away. But the light from the overhead streetlight had allowed J.P. to see the glistening in Arthur's eyes.

He also remembered the nights that he and Arthur had sat up until two or three in the morning talking. Sean had gone to his house, and J.P. had stayed a while. They talked about things that would have seemed totally unimportant to anyone listening in on the conversation, but they were important to him, and he was sure they were important to Arthur. They talked about the way girls were today, and the way they were when Arthur had grown up in the sixties. They talked of many things on many nights. None of the things they talked about would bring world peace or

136

make the world a better place in which to live in, but those conversations that he had with Arthur made his small part of the world a better place for him to live J.P. would miss his friends, too. They had become a major part of his life. A life that would never be the same again.

The reality of the present tore his thoughts from the memories of the past.

"Show us the place where Arthur fell," he said softly.

"Follow me," Mark answered. It would not have done any good to argue with either of them.

****

Thomas stood in the woods just out of their sight as they rode past him. Killing them was not going to be easy. But it would not be too difficult, either. They thought he was dead, so they would become careless. He would wait for the right moment and then his woods would be safe again.

Thomas knew that they would have to pass him on the way out of the woods. There was no need for him to follow them up the hill. He had a few things to take care of before they tried to leave the woods anyway.

****

Tiffanie felt the cold, rough hands grab her and drag her from the truck as the water almost covered her face. She barely felt the pain as she was dropped on the asphalt road. In the beginning, she tried to resist, but it was useless and she gave up and let herself be taken. Her strength was gone, as well as her will to survive.

Tiffanie then slipped into unconsciousness, closed her mind, and isolated her feelings from the world around her. There was peace and quiet in the darkness. At this moment, she craved that peace more than anything else in the world.

****

The rain stopped just as they topped the hill and drove over to the edge of the other side.

"He went over right here," Mark said as he pointed downward.

Sean looked over the cliff and saw the tops of the pine trees. His eyes followed the trail of broken branches as far as his vision would allow him. The distance was so great that he could not see all the way to the ground. His heart tried to harbor a hope, but his brain forced the logic through and the hope in his heart changed to sadness. His father was dead, and it was his fault. If he and J.P. had not gotten lost and had returned sooner, on time, Arthur would not have tried to kill the old man for revenge. His father was dead because he was late, just as he always was. Sean searched his confused mind for the answer his father had asked him a thousand times over the years. Why was he always late? Why couldn't he get somewhere at the time he said he would? Sean also wondered about the answer to another question that came into his mind as he looked over the steep cliff. Why hadn't he listened to his father over the years? It seemed that his father was always griping at him for being late. The griping had always gotten on his nerves in the past, but at this moment, he would give anything if he could have heard his dad give him the ass-chewing of his life. He would not have ignored it this time as he always had before. He would have listened to every word his father said. He would have smiled as his father lectured on the importance of being punctual. He would have hugged his father as tightly as he could instead of rolling his eyes as he had done in the past.

Sean made a solemn promise to himself that he would never be late for anything again as long as he lived. If he went to a wedding, he would be so early that he would get there before the bride did. That would make his father proud, though it would not help him now. He hoped that somehow his father would know. Wherever his father's soul was now, he hoped that he would know.

The three of them stood in silence looking over the cliff and down into the space below. Each of them was lost in his own thoughts as they recalled fond memories of the times they had spent with Arthur.

J.P. remembered the time Arthur and he had replaced the transmission on the Mustang. As the memory came to him, he wished that he had not complained about working on Fords as much as he had. He hoped that he had not hurt Arthur's feelings. He remembered how hard Arthur had tried to help with the work on the car. Most of the time he had only been in the way, and J.P. had to work around him. Arthur was not much of a mechanic, but he had refused to stand around and watch idly while someone else did all the work. That was the kind of man he was. J.P. wished that they could work on something together again. He wished for it more than anything else in the world even though he knew it was impossible. If he could get his wish, he wouldn't even object if it were a Ford.

As he looked over the cliff, Mark remembered the time he had stayed at Arthur's home when he had no electricity in his apartment in the middle of winter. Arthur had insisted that it was too cold for him to stay at his apartment. It would have been easier for Arthur to loan him the money to get the power turned back on, but he didn't do that. Not because he was cheap or stingy, but because he wanted to let Mark know that he had to make his own way in life and he had to take the responsibility of paying his own way. Arthur had also shown him that he had someone to depend on if he got a little behind on those responsibilities. Because of Arthur, Mark had learned those lessons well and he would never forget them. He would never forget Arthur, either. Mark made up his mind that he would do his best to be the type of father Arthur was.

Sean did not wipe the tears away as they streamed down his face. He did not care if J.P. and Mark saw him cry. This was not a time for manly pride. This was a time to remember the man who was lying at the bottom of this cliff. A man who had always been there for him throughout his entire life. A man who sacrificed everything for his family. His dad was a man who was always there for him whenever he needed him. He was never too busy to answer stupid questions or listen to unimportant problems. He and his dad did not always agree on everything, but at least his father listened to his side. Sean remembered the man lying at the bottom of the cliff teaching him to ride a bicycle and how to drive a stick shift car. That man had always displayed the patience of a saint. He would miss that man more than he could ever imagine. Sean would miss the man who had been on the sidelines at every Judo and Karate tournament he had ever fought, cheering louder than any other parent. Sean regretted every minute he had caused his father to worry. He regretted a lot of things. Things that he would never have the opportunity to change now. He could never replace the man who was always there when he needed him.

****

Thomas took his position in the woods. They would be coming this way in a few minutes. He knew exactly what he was going to do. They would not separate, so he was going to have to take them all at the same time. It would not be as easy to take three of them at the same time, so he would have to eliminate one of them quickly. It still would not be easy to kill the remaining two, at least not as simple as it was to kill the two sissies. All three of these were strong, and, once they discovered that he was still alive, they would have their sagging spirits renewed with a passionate hatred that would make them braver than they would normally be. It could give them the power to kill him. Thomas could tell by the silence of the woods that they were still on the top of the hill. He sat on the ground and leaned against a tall pine tree that lined the trail. It would not be very long before they would be coming this way. He closed his eyes and relaxed.

****

"We can't just leave him down there," Sean said as he went to the edge.

"What are you going to do?" J.P. asked as he joined him.

"I'm going to climb down there and stay with him until Tiffanie comes back with the cops."

"You're crazy! You can't climb down there! You'll fall and kill yourself!" J.P. argued.

"I can't let him just lay down there on the ground all alone."

"There's nothing you can do for him now," J.P. consoled Sean.

"I don't give a damn about that! I have to get to him!" Sean yelled as he pushed J.P. away and slipped over the edge of the cliff.

Mark and J.P. grabbed his arms and pulled him back to the top.

"It's suicide to try and get to him this way!" Mark said as he held on to Sean's arm.

J.P. held the other one.

"I can make it. There are a few toeholds on the rocks."

"No, you can't! Are you trying to kill yourself?" J.P. yelled in his face.

"What else is there to live for?"

"What about your mother?" J.P. asked. "How am I going to tell her that you broke your neck for no reason? She is going to suffer enough grief as it is. Do you want to double that grief?"

Sean stopped struggling to release himself from their grip. J.P. was right. His mother would need him now more than ever since his father was gone. She would never get over his death, and he didn't want to add to her burdens.

"All right. I can't go down that way. But I'm still not going to leave him down there," Sean said.

"We don't to leave him either. Look over there," J.P. said.

Sean and Mark looked in the direction J.P. was pointing. It was a small hill opposite the one they were standing on. They squinted and saw the small trail leading down the side of the hill to the bottom.

"We can reach him from there. It might be a little tricky, but we can do it," J.P. continued.

"All right. Let's go. It will be dark soon," Sean said.

****

Thomas heard the noise of the engines and opened his eyes. He had fallen asleep, and the riders were almost upon him.

He swung his stick as the first one passed, it was the one he had heard the other ones call Sean. The stick connected and hit him across the chest as he passed. The rider went backwards off the motorcycle and landed on his back.

Thomas didn't have time to draw his stick back so he let the second rider pass. As the third rider went by he shoved the stick between the spokes in the front wheel and the rider went flying over the front of the motorcycle and fell near the first rider.

The speed the motorcycle was going, combined with the force of being jammed between the spokes, jerked the stick from Thomas's hand. He ran as fast as he could to retrieve it.

He looked over his shoulder and saw that the three were not hurt badly. He grabbed his stick and went into the woods.

Mark saw Sean fall in front of him and swerved to avoid running over him. He barely missed rolling over his head as he slammed on his brakes, stopped, and ran over to Sean. He caught a glimpse of Thomas as he caused J.P. to wreck.

J.P. hit the ground and was on his feet immediately helping Mark with Sean. He had taken much worse spills in all his years of riding motorcycles.

He was relieved to see that Sean was all right. The blow from the stick had just knocked the breath out of him.

Mark and J.P. picked Sean up. He was trying to breathe.

"Are you all right?" Mark asked him.

After a few quick, deep breaths Sean answered. "I think I've got a hell of a bruise, but I'm all right."

"Thank God for chest plates," J.P. said as he tapped the steel chest through Sean's jacket.

"What the hell happened?" Sean asked.

"It was him. The old man that killed the others," Mark answered.

"I thought you said he was dead."

"I saw him go off the cliff with your dad. Maybe he grabbed hold of something and caught himself. Or maybe he can't die," Mark said.

"He can die, and the bastard will, too," Sean said as his face turned red with anger and hatred for the old man.

"What do we do now? He'll be waiting for us at every turn in the trail on the way out," J.P. said. "We may not be so lucky next time. Sooner or later he will get one of us, maybe even all of us."

"I don't know about you two. But I'm not going to wait for him to get me," Sean answered. "I'm going after him."

J.P. went to his motorcycle and picked it up and checked the front wheel. There were a few spokes missing, but it was still drivable.

"I'm going with you," J.P. said. "I'll be damned if he is going to kill my friends and get away with it."

"Count me in, too," Mark said.

"Good. I know for a fact that this trail makes a circle around the woods he went into. I rode over it several times today. Mark, you go to the left. J.P., you go to the right. He has to come out somewhere. One of us is bound to spot him. Whenever one of us does, yell as loud as you can."

"Where are you going?" Mark asked.

"I'll cut through the woods. He won't know which way to go."

No more words were spoken as each of them went in a different direction. There were no words to describe the way they felt. The three of them were not afraid anymore. They were angry now. Their anger was so great that it overrode any fear that they might have had. They had a mission now. Their anger was reinforced by a pride that they would not run away. They were willing to stand and fight. If they died trying to complete that mission, that was all right with them. It was better to die standing tall like a man fighting rather than cringing in fear and being afraid of every movement they saw on the way out of the woods. Movement might be caused by a falling pine needle blown by the wind, or a rabbit scurrying out of the way of the noise of their motorcycles. Life was precious to them, and they held that value dearly. But so was their pride, and without that pride, there could be no meaningful life.

143

****

Thomas watched them from the woods. He heard every single word they said. The expressions on their faces told him that he had to get back to his bunker. Their determination, as well as their hatred for Thomas, would be to their advantage. He would let these three go. They would not violate his woods again. He was certain of that. As the three took off, so did he.

Thomas ran through the woods. Another hundred feet and he would be at the bottom of the hill that he had to climb to get to his bunker.

The sound of the motorcycle bearing down upon him told him he would not make it. He turned and held his stick firmly in his hand and raised it high as the rider stopped and threw his motorcycle to the ground. The rider stopped ten feet in front of him. Just out of the range of the stick.

They stared at each other for a full minute before the rider finally spoke. "You killed my father."

"I've killed many people. They all deserved to die."

"He didn't. You didn't even know him. You didn't know the kind of man he was," Sean accused.

"It doesn't matter. He trespassed in my woods. For that he had to die. Just as the others did who trespassed in my woods."

"This is Government property."

"This is my property. They stole it from my father," Thomas said with strong emotion.

"I don't give a damn who it belongs to. You had no right to kill my father or anyone else."

Thomas tightened his grip on the stick.

"I didn't kill your father."

"You caused his death!" Sean screamed.

"We all must do what we have to do," Thomas answered.

"That's the only thing we will ever agree on," Sean said as he ran toward Thomas.

Thomas waited until he was close enough before he swung his stick. He swung it harder than he ever had before. Sean ducked and slammed his body into Thomas with a force that sent him reeling backward and sprawling to the ground. He looked up and Sean was standing over him.

"Get up!" Sean yelled.

Thomas stood up and tightened his grip on his stick even more although it would not be of much use to him now. Sean was standing too close to be hit with it.

"Are you ready to die?"

"Are you ready to kill me?" Thomas laughed. He was bigger than this young man. Once he got his hands on him, he would crush him. He dropped the stick and waited for the opportunity to finish off this brash young man.

Sean spun around and brought his foot high into the air and kicked Thomas hard on the side of his head. The blow made Thomas move backward a few steps, but he did not fall.

"Is that the best you can do?"

Sean answered the question with another kick that caught Thomas in the groin. He doubled over and fell to his knees. Sean didn't wait for him to recover. He pounded him in the face over and over again until his knuckles bled and his blood mixed with the blood that flowed from Thomas's face.

Sean stopped his attack when he was totally out of breath. He looked at Thomas. He was still on his knees. He spun around again and landed a hard, swift kick in the center of Thomas's chest that sent him backward again. This time he did not get up.

J.P. and Mark rode up and threw down their bikes. They stood with their fists clenched, hatred in their eyes, and revenge on their minds. They were ready to fight.

Sean smiled as he walked away from Thomas.

"Is he dead?" Mark asked.

"No. I don't know why, but I couldn't bring myself to kill him. I wanted to. I just couldn't do it."

"I don't think your father would have wanted you to do it. Not when it wasn't necessary," J.P. said in a low voice as he tried to control the almost overwhelming urge within him that wanted to choke the life out of Thomas.

"Maybe you're right," Sean said.

"I know I'm right."

145

"Well, he may not be dead, but he is going to be hurting a lot when he wakes up," Sean said as he stared at Thomas.

Mark walked over and looked down at Thomas.

"He doesn't look so dangerous now. He looks like exactly what he is, an old man. He looks so harmless."

"Try telling that to all the others. It won't do any good, they can't hear you," J.P. said.

"I need a cigarette. Then we'll find something to tie him up with. Afterward, we can go find my dad," Sean said as he walked away from Thomas. It disgusted him to look at him. He also didn't trust himself not to kill Thomas anyway if he woke up too soon.

The three of them walked back over to Sean's bike and waited as he opened the small pouch that was fastened to his seat. He handed each of them a cigarette. He lit his own and Mark's. He was about to hand J.P. the lighter out of habit when J.P. leaned his head forward and put the cigarette that he held between his lips near the lighter as Sean lit it. He took a deep drag from it and blew the smoke out.

"It's kind of funny," he said. "but little things that used to bother me a lot don't seem that important anymore."

"Don't expect me to be opening doors for you for the rest of your life," Mark joked.

Their laughter seemed out of place in their surroundings. But it was a welcome relief to the sadness that had occupied the last few hours.

"Stop, put it down," a voice to the side of them shouted.

The sound of a gun exploding caused a ringing in their ears as they turned and saw Thomas standing right behind them with his stick over his head ready to attack them.

A stream of blood flowed from his chest and covered the front of his shirt as he released his grip on the stick, and it fell harmlessly to the ground. He stared at them with a hatred in his eyes as he fell face forward on the ground.

"It looks like we got here just in time," the State Policeman dressed in a blue uniform said as he returned his gun to his holster.

Sean, J.P., and Mark watched as the huge State Policeman

146

who would make a pro football player look like a dwarf walked over to Thomas and used his boot to roll him over on his back.

"He looks dead to me, but you boys had better check him anyway," he said to the two paramedics who had come into the woods with him.

"Who wants to tell me what the Hell is going on?" he asked as he spit out a big wad of tobacco and walked over to them.

They all started speaking at once, and he put his hand up.

"I can't understand a word any of you are saying. Which one of you is Mark?"

Mark raised his hand as if he were in school and wanted to ask permission to go to the bathroom.

"Okay, Mark. I'm Officer Wayne Trahan. Tell me the story."

"Is Tiffanie all right?"

"She'll be fine. A few cuts and bruises from the accident, but she'll recover."

"What accident?"

"She slid the truck off the road into a ditch. It was lucky for her she had the headlights on and a motorist passing by the main road saw them or she would have drowned in that ditch. It's too bad she wasn't so lucky when the paramedics arrived. That clumsy dumb ass over there dropped her on the road and broke her arm. If I were her, I'd sue the piss out of him."

The paramedic who had dropped Tiffanie started to say something, but changed his mind.

"Did she tell you that she was pregnant? Is the baby okay?" Mark asked.

"She told us. The baby is fine. She also told us that there were bodies all over the place in these woods. We found two on the trail here. Are there any more?"

"Lots of them," Mark answered.

"Did he kill them all?"

"Yes," Sean interrupted Mark before he could answer. "He said he was protecting his woods."

"I've heard stories about that guy. I thought it was all a bunch of crap. There's not much for the people that live around here to do except make up stories since the base closed. I guess I was wrong," Officer Trahan said.

"Dead wrong," J.P. said.

"Are there any more of you unaccounted for?" the policeman asked.

"No."

"Then there's not much left to do. I called on the radio for backup. They should be here soon. We'll look for all the bodies and haul them out then."

"I've got to find my dad."

"I thought you said everyone was accounted for."

"His dad went off a cliff on his motorcycle," J.P. said as he lowered his gaze toward the ground.

"I'm going to find him anyway."

"I don't blame you, son. I would want to do the same thing if I were in your shoes. Do you have any idea where he landed?" the policeman asked.

"Yes."

"Good. I'll go with you. Ride me on the back of your motorcycle until we get to that bunker over the next hill. I can pick up the bike in there. Those two boys won't be needing it anymore," Officer Trahan stated.

****

Arthur opened his eyes and saw the gray sky hovering above him through the branches of the trees. He wondered for an instant if he were dead. He decided he wasn't because his arms hurt. The blood oozing from the corner of his mouth told him that he had sustained some serious injuries in the fall. He tried to move his legs, but they did not respond. He could not even feel them. He couldn't even move his hands to see if they were still there. They could have been shorn off by the jagged limbs on the way down.

As he lay on the ground, he wondered why he hadn't been killed. As he looked far above him, he found the answer to that question. The hundreds of tree branches he had fallen through had slowed him enough that he did not hit the ground at full

148

impact. He was thankful that one of the branches had knocked him out on the way down, and he did not have to see the ground as it came toward him. Arthur was thankful for something else, too. He was thankful that God had given him a few more minutes of life to ask for forgiveness for all the mistakes he had made in his life.

Arthur knew that the injuries he had sustained in the fall had to be bad. Death was certainly only a short period of time away. He decided to spend part of that time praying. The rest of the time he had left until Death dropped its shroud over him would be spent remembering the good times he had experienced in his lifetime.

****

James Foster woke up. "How could I have fallen asleep in such a place?" he asked himself as he looked at the occupant of the cage he was tied to. It must have been the booze, he thought, or because he had stayed up all night. Whatever the reason was, it was not important now. The important thing was that he had to get himself loose and out of this place before the old man came back. The thought of seeing him again did not appeal to James.

He jerked and tugged at the vines that bound his hands. They were too strong to break. They were wrapped around his wrists so tightly that he could not loosen them at all. He leaned his head toward the cage and tried to bite them. The occupant of the cage slammed into the wire and he pulled his head away. That would not work, either. The wire that formed the cage was the type with huge squares. If the occupant got the opportunity to take a bite out of him, he would lose at least a finger. James decided to continue trying to break the vines by rubbing them back and forth along the wire.

****

Arthur finished his final prayers and let his mind wander. He thought of Elizabeth and the first time they met. It was love at first sight, and he had never wanted to make love to another woman since that time. Before he met her he went after every woman he could. He had stored his conquests of women in his mind the way that hunters collected trophies. The sight of her had changed all of that. He was glad when she resisted his advances to make love to her. She was only fifteen years old then, but possessed the wisdom of a woman far beyond her years. She understood that a woman must respect herself in order for a man to respect her.

Arthur also remembered the two years they had dated. Those memories helped to ease the pain in his arms that began to spread to other parts of his body.

Arthur concentrated on his memories even more to shut out the pain. He summoned a picture of Elizabeth in her wedding gown. She was so beautiful that night, and her beauty had grown with the passing years. He remembered the glow that seemed to surround her when she was pregnant. He remembered her slightly crooked smile that always brought a warm feeling to his entire being. Elizabeth was one of a kind, and he was the luckiest man in the world for the time he had spent with her. A twinge of sadness overcame him as he remembered something he had jokingly told her a few weeks ago. He had told her that if anything ever happened to him that he didn't want her to remarry. He told her that he would come back from the dead and hover over her if she slept with another man. Many wives would have gotten angry if their husbands had said that to them. Elizabeth had smiled and said that there would never be another man for her. And he knew she meant it. Now, as he lay dying, he regretted telling her that. She was still a young woman who had the rest of her life ahead of her. It would be such a waste, especially with Sean also gone, if she had to spend the rest of her life alone.

A fierce pain broke through his memories and began to wrack his body. He spit up a clump of blood that fell on his chest, and he knew that his time was growing short. There was also no way he could tell Elizabeth that his last thoughts were of her. Even if he had a pen and paper, he could not move his arms to write her a note. He hoped and prayed that he had told her enough how much he loved her. If he hadn't, that was something that he would have to carry to his grave along with his other regrets. Those regrets included the reality that he would never spend another cold night in front of the fireplace with her sipping coffee laced with Irish Creme, or slow dancing with her by the crackling fire to the soft sound of music by Percy Sledge. Their favorite was "When a Man Loves a Woman." Arthur knew that to sing it with such feeling the way he did, Percy had to have experienced that kind of love. He hoped that Percy and his wife were safe and together at this very moment. He hoped that they were sharing the kind of love that he and Elizabeth could never share again.

Arthur held his breath and waited until another sharp pain in his chest subsided before he returned to his memories. He remembered holding his children for the first time. He tried to remember, who was the oldest? Was it his daughter April? His mind was becoming like the sky above him. A hazy grey. He used all his will to concentrate. No, April was the youngest. Chad was the oldest, and Sean was in the middle. "Yes," He said aloud. That was right. April had to work the night he left, and he had not even said goodbye. He regretted it now that he hadn't gone to the grocery store where she worked and kissed her goodbye one last time. Arthur tried to remember the last time he saw Chad. Was it last week at Christmas? No, he remembered now. Chad was working out of state and did not get to come home for Christmas. It must have been at least a month, he reasoned. As hard as he tried, Arthur could not remember the last words he had said to his oldest son. That fact saddened him greatly.

The sky above him, like his memory, grew darker as he remembered holding his granddaughters. Nicole was Chad's daughter. Elise and Ashton were Sean's. They were beautiful little girls who filled his life with many hours of pleasure. Arthur was filled with added disappointment when he thought of his only grandson, Chance. Chance was the sole heir to carry on the family name. Arthur shed a single tear because he would never get to know Chance. He would miss them all. He hoped that Elizabeth would tell them about him as they grew older. He hoped that she would tell them how much he loved them. He felt very secure in the knowledge that she would. Arthur thought about his parents for a moment. He would miss them, too. They were special people who always did their best to show all their children the same love and understanding he had shown his children. Arthur wished that he could tell them thank you for the values they had instilled in him that shaped his life before he died. He couldn't remember if he ever had before.

Arthur allowed his mind to wander freely. It led to thoughts of his older brother, Chris. He and Arthur had planned a fishing trip for next month. They had planned it down to the very last detail to make sure everything went perfectly. Arthur realized how unfair death could be. It could wreck even the best laid plans.

As he felt a coldness come over him, Arthur remembered the good times he and his brother had growing up. Arthur was like Chris' shadow. Everywhere Chris went, Arthur was right behind him asking dumb questions and wanting to know what they were going to do tomorrow. Chris had always told him to live for today, tomorrow would take care of itself. Arthur knew as he lay on the wet pine straw that there would be no tomorrow for him.

Arthur closed his eyes and formed a picture of Elizabeth in his mind. He could not think anymore. He wanted to die with the vision of her in his mind. Elizabeth's face was the last thing he wanted to see as his soul passed from this world to the next one.

****

James Foster continued pulling on the vines attached to the cage until he was exhausted. He lay on his side and rested.

"There has to be some way out of this," he said as he studied the vines that were wrapped around the wire.

He looked past the vines and followed the wire. His heart almost jumped from his chest with excitement. Why hadn't he seen it before? There was only one metal staple that connected the wire to the wooden part of the bottom of the cage. If he could break the strands of wire below the section where the vines that held him were tied, he could pull the rusted staple out and he would be free. He cursed himself for not seeing it sooner. He blamed that on the effects of the alcohol, too.

James slammed his wrists in a downward motion and after several tries the first wire broke free. There were only three below it that he would have to break before he would be able to pull the staple.

The occupant of the cage sat quietly in the corner staring at him.

****

Arthur heard the sounds of the forest at night and opened his eyes. An owl sat in the tree above him and hooted, and a bullfrog in the distance croaked.

Arthur heard the sounds of twigs snapping and managed to turn his head to the direction of the sound. The way his luck was going today, it would probably be a wolf or some other animal that would eat him alive. That didn't seem fair to him. When he and Elizabeth went out for dinner, he would not even pick out the lobster he wanted to eat from a large aquarium. He always told the waiter that he did not want to get on speaking terms with his meal before he ate it. Now he was going to be eaten by something that would not return the kindness he had shown the lobsters.

The sounds grew nearer as he stared into the darkness and wondered what his fate was going to be. Through the darkness he saw one eye of the animal. This was even more humiliating. He was going to be eaten by a one-eyed wolf. He stifled a laugh. It hurt too much.

The eye became larger as it got closer him and Arthur realized that it was not an eye at all. It was a light. A single light that pierced through the darkness. Arthur remembered seeing something on television about people who had been brought back from the brink of death. They all told the same story. Each of them talked about a bright light that shined out of the darkness. None of them could say what was behind the light because they were revived at the last possible moment before they reached that light. Arthur stared at the light. He would know very soon what the people on the television show did not. He would see the other side of the light.

"Here he is! I found him!" the State Policeman yelled.

Arthur saw the big man holding the flashlight.

"I hope this doesn't hurt your feelings," Arthur said, "but you are the ugliest angel I've ever seen."

"How many have you seen?" the policeman asked.

"Counting you?" Arthur asked.

"Yes."

"You're the first."

"Good. Then you don't have anything to compare me to."

Arthur didn't have time to respond. Sean came around the policeman and dropped to the ground next to him and reached for the father he thought he had lost.

"Hold on a minute, son," the policeman said as he stopped Sean from touching Arthur. "We don't know what all is wrong with him. You don't want to do any more damage than what's been done by the fall from that cliff up there."

Arthur smiled at Sean. He was alive. He should have known it all along. Sean was a survivor.

"It's okay, son. I'm going to be all right, now that you are here."

Sean slid his hand across the wet pine straw and touched his father's hand lightly and looked into his eyes. He was so happy and so engrossed in the moment that he didn't even hear the policeman's booming voice as he yelled to the paramedics.

"Get your asses over here fast. Can't you see there is an injured man here?"

Very little was said between Sean and Arthur during the time it took for the paramedics to check him over and place splints on almost every part of his body. They eased him onto a stretcher just as the helicopter from the hospital hovered overhead and shined a spotlight down on them. It lit up the entire area.

"Your father is a lucky man," one of the paramedics said to Sean. "That fall should have killed him."

"Is he going to be all right?"

"Both his legs and arms are broken, and he certainly has

some internal injuries, but the sooner we get him to the hospital, the better his chances will be. He's tough. He survived that fall. I think he just might make it."

"That is, if they don't drop him," the State Trooper said.

The helicopter lowered a cable with two hooks connected to the end of it and the paramedics attached a hook to each end of the stretcher.

"Are you ready?" the policeman asked.

"Just a second," Arthur answered.

He motioned with his head for Sean, Mark and J.P. to come over to his side.

"Do you three want to go riding next weekend?" Arthur asked them.

"You better plan on a little longer than that," the paramedic said.

"I'll be ready when you are," Sean said as he brushed a tear away.

"Me, too," Mark agreed.

"Don't worry about it, Mr. Billings, I mean, Dad," J.P. said. "It will take me at least that long to fix your motorcycle. You are really going to have to learn to be more careful."

"You boys sure know how to bring in the New Year," Arthur said as he felt a pain go through his chest.

"You think this one was strange? Wait until you see what we've planned for next year," Sean said as he grinned.

"*I can wait*."

The paramedic gave a signal to the helicopter pilot and he slowly began to lift the stretcher from the ground.

"Put some mud tires on that thing when you fix it, J.P. Sean will pay for them," Arthur said as the helicopter carried him high into the air until the stretcher cleared the treetops. Then it flew away.

CHAPTER 14

James Foster broke though the remaining wires and pulled with all the strength he could get from his tired body to free the staple that held him prisoner. He managed to get his feet around and use them as he strained against the cage.

He fell backward as the staple loosened and finally came out. He looked around the bunker in the dim light of the fire. That madman must have a knife around here somewhere. He stopped his search when he heard the sound behind him. The occupant of the cage was crawling out. When he had removed the staple, James had also made an area between the frame of the cage and the wire large enough for the occupant to crawl through.

James backed up several feet. The occupant of the cage stood up. He was almost as tall as James was. James got a good look at what had been locked up in the cage for the first time. He was so much larger than he seemed to be when he was in a crouching position.

"Let's talk this over. I did you a favor by letting you out of that cage," James said.

The only answer James received was a low growl as the occupant lunged at him and tore out his throat. He fell to the floor as the blood gushed from the wound. He watched with terror in his eyes as the occupant bit him in the stomach and began eating his insides. It was only a matter of moments until James's screams fell silent.

****

He stood in the safety of the trees and watched the policemen as they loaded the last body into the ambulance. That was the body of Thomas, his father. He felt no sadness as he saw the blood covered shirt or the cold stare of death on his face. He felt only relief that he was free.

He had no idea how long Thomas had kept him locked in that cage. Time meant nothing to him. It was just a way of measuring the distance between the time the sun set and rose again.

He had stopped counting the days, weeks, and months long ago. His memory was vivid of the day that Thomas had first brought him and his mother to these woods. Thomas had tried to explain to them that both his wife and son belonged with him. He and his mother had tried to escape Thomas many times, but he always caught them and brought them back and beat them. The last time they had escaped, Thomas had beaten his mother to death and had put him in the cage. Thomas was so angry with him that he put his mother's body in the cage with him and told him to eat her when he got hungry. Thomas had shouted and tormented him with food so much that one day his hunger overcame his love for his mother, and he did eat her. He ate every part of her he could, and he enjoyed it. Afterward, he was riddled with guilt, and Thomas had explained how everything goes back into the earth and gets reborn. Thomas kept him locked in the cage so he would not escape again. His father would not believe him when he pleaded to be let out and promised he would not try to escape again. He had stopped pleading long ago. He had also stopped talking. His time was spent listening to Thomas constantly telling him, since the first day he put him the cage, that these woods would be his one day. Thomas always said that after he was dead, the burden of protecting the woods would fall on his shoulders. It was such a heavy burden that it would take a person that was part man, and part animal to carry out the duties that such a burden placed on the man who undertook it. That was one of the reasons he ate his meat raw. He wanted to protect the woods. He learned to growl like an animal so he could strike fear in the hearts of anyone that came into the woods. With his mother dead, and now Thomas, the only thing he had left in his life was these woods.

As he watched the ambulance drive away, he smiled. He would let them go this time. They could take the remains of their dead away from here. They were not worthy of being returned to his earth anyway. But if they came back again, he would be waiting for them, and they would not leave his woods alive a second time.

He was Thomas' son. That made him the "Keeper of the Woods" now, and no one had better ever forget it. *He would not be as kind to trespassers as Thomas had been.*

Chester A. "Chet" Ballard is a resident of Denham Springs, Louisiana.

Previously released novels by Chester A. "Chet" Ballard

Stalker
Dark Visions

About the Author

Chester A. Ballard resides in Denham Springs, Louisiana, with his wife of twenty-nine years. They have three children. Mr. Ballard has worked in many occupations, and went back to school to get a degree in computer programming. He continued on in this line of work until his wife convinced him to give it up for his true passion—writing. Since then, he has completed nine novels and started eight more. His two published works are "Stalker," and "Dark Visions." This is his first novel with 1st Books.